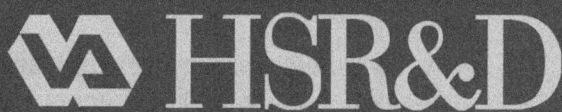

I0470827

Assessment and Management of Acute Pain in Adult Medical Inpatients: A Systematic Review

April 2008

Prepared for:

Department of Veterans Affairs
Veterans Health Administration
Health Services Research & Development Service
Washington, DC 20420

Investigators:

Mark Helfand, MD, MPH
Director

Michele Freeman, MPH
Research Associate

Prepared by:

Portland Veterans Affairs Healthcare System
Oregon Evidence-based Practice Center
Portland, OR

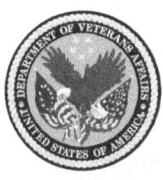

PREFACE

VA's Health Services Research and Development Service (HSR&D) works to improve the cost, quality, and outcomes of health care for our nation's veterans. Collaborating with VA leaders, managers, and policy makers, HSR&D focuses on important health care topics that are likely to have significant impact on quality improvement efforts. One significant collaborative effort is HSR&D's Evidence-based Synthesis Program (ESP). Through this program, HSR&D provides timely and accurate evidence syntheses on targeted health care topics. These products will be disseminated broadly throughout VA and will: inform VA clinical policy, develop clinical practice guidelines, set directions for future research to address gaps in knowledge, identify the evidence to support VA performance measures, and rationalize drug formulary decisions.

HSR&D provided funding for the two Evidence Based Practice Centers (EPCs) supported by the Agency for Healthcare Research and Quality (AHRQ) that also had an active and publicly acknowledged VA affiliation—Southern California EPC and Portland, OR EPC—so they could develop evidence syntheses on requested topics for dissemination to VA policymakers. A planning committee with representation from HSR&D, Patient Care Services, Office of Quality and Performance, and the VISN Clinical Management Officers, has been established to identify priority topics and to ensure the quality of final reports. Comments on this evidence report are welcome and can be sent to Susan Schiffner, ESP Program Manager, at Susan.Schiffner@va.gov.

EXECUTIVE SUMMARY

BACKGROUND

Poor pain management in surgical settings is known to be associated with slower recovery, greater morbidity, longer lengths of stay, lower patient satisfaction, and higher costs of care, suggesting that optimal pain care in these settings is of utmost importance in promoting acute illness management, recovery, and adaptation. VA/DoD Clinical Practice Guidelines have been developed for the management of acute post-operative pain, although the basis for many of the recommendations was by expert consensus rather than empirical evidence.

The prevalence of pain on the inpatient medical ward is lower than that of a surgical service, but is still substantial. In one hospital survey, 43% of medical ward patients experienced pain, and 12% reported unbearable pain. There are currently no pain-relevant performance measures in place that can support efforts to enhance pain care in these settings, and research on pain management in nonsurgical, nonmalignant acute pain is sparse.

The Key Questions were:

1. For inpatients who have acute pain, how do differences in timing and frequency of assessment, severity of pain, and follow-up of pain affect choice of treatment, clinical outcomes, and safety?

2. How do the timing and route of administration of pain interventions compare in effectiveness, adverse effects, and safety in these inpatient care settings?

3. For inpatients with impaired self-report due to any of several factors, including delirium or confusion, pre-existing severe dementia, closed head injury, stroke, and psychosis, how do differences in assessment and management of acute pain affect clinical outcomes or safety?

4. For inpatients with dependencies on tobacco, alcohol, stimulant, marijuana, or opioids, how do differences in assessment and management of acute pain affect clinical outcomes or safety? How do the assessment and management of acute pain differ between patients on prexisting opioid therapy and patients with opiate addiction?

METHODS

We searched in Medline (via PubMed), PubMed Clinical Queries, and the Cochrane Database of Systematic Reviews (searched via EBM) for systematic reviews published from 1996 to April, 2007. We also conducted a focused search in Medline for primary studies published from 1950 to July 2007 that address KQ1 or the use of PCA for non-surgical pain. Additional citations were identified from reference lists and searches of web sites devoted to pain management. Two investigators independently reviewed titles, abstracts, and articles, and performed a critical analysis of the literature and compiled narrative summaries to address the key questions.

RESULTS

We screened 3069 titles and abstracts, and performed a more detailed review on 211 articles. From these, we identified recent systematic reviews, randomized controlled trials (RCTs), and observational studies that addressed one of the key questions.

Key Question #1 Timing and Frequency, Severity, and Followup

<u>Evidence in Target Population</u>
No evidence that directly linked the timing, frequency, or choice of measure for assessment with the timeliness, choice, or safety of treatment specifically in medical inpatients. The psychometric properties of different pain intensity measures in hospitalized patients with nonsurgical, noncancer pain is not known. There are no good-quality studies comparing different assessment methods in the general medical inpatient setting.

There is good evidence that treating abdominal pain does not compromise timely diagnosis and treatment of the surgical abdomen.

<u>Relevant Evidence from Other Settings</u>
There is fair evidence from case series about the psychometric properties of different pain intensity measures in the outpatient, postsurgical, and palliative care settings. However, this evidence is not likely to be applicable to medical inpatients.

In the emergency department, patients who have mild to moderate pain that is not due to malignancy or coronary disease receive less timely, and less effective treatment than other patients. This finding is likely to be relevant to inpatients as well. Potential risk factors for delayed or inadequate analgesia include female sex, less severe pain, and daytime admissions. Crowding in the ER is also associated with undertreatment of pain.

Key Question #2 Timing and Route of Administration of Pain Medications

<u>Evidence in Target Population</u>

There is fair evidence from one randomized trial that a multifaceted institutional intervention improved assessment and increased analgesic prescribing, but the intervention did not alter severity of pain. We found no evidence about the value of coordinating care with the patient's primary care physician.

Patient-controlled analgesia is used with increasing frequency in medical patients, but its safety and effectiveness have not been studied in this setting.

<u>Relevant Evidence from Other Settings</u>

In a good-quality systematic review of 32 studies, institutional interventions improved pain assessment and documentation and staff awareness of pain, and increased use of analgesics. While pain management teams and other system-wide interventions improved the timeliness and frequency of pain assessment, the findings were mixed for improvement in pain outcomes. In controlled studies, Acute Pain Services reduced pain intensity and improved functional ability, although the magnitude of these effects was not always clinically important.

After surgery, patients using PCA consume higher amounts of opioids and have better pain control and higher satisfaction than patients treated with prn or scheduled opioid treatments, with no higher incidence of most side effects. However, the effectiveness of safety of PCA in nonsurgical, nonmalignant acute pain is not known.

Key Question #3 Patients with Impaired Self-report

There is weak evidence that most cognitively impaired individuals can understand at least one self-assessment measure. For patients who cannot understand any of the self-assessment measures, some guidelines recommend use of an observational assessment measure, while others recommend empiric pain treatment if the impaired patient has diagnoses usually associated with pain. Almost no evidence is available to guide management of pain in delirium.

Key Question #4 Patients with drug dependencies

Several instruments intended to screen chronic opioid users for addiction may be helpful in assessing whether relevant signs, symptoms, and behaviors are present. Evidence about treating pain in patients with substance abuse disorders or chronic opioid use is weak, being derived from case reports, retrospective studies and expert opinion.

TABLE OF CONTENTS

INTRODUCTION

"With the exception of the PACU, the floor will be the most common place where hospitalized patients may need acute pain management." [1]

Many guidelines and previous reviews address pain assessment and management in surgical inpatients, trauma patients, inpatients with cancer, and inpatients with sickle cell crisis. In contrast, pain in medical inpatients with other conditions has received little attention. The prevalence of pain on the inpatient medical ward is lower than that of a surgical service, but is still substantial. In one hospital survey, 43% of medical ward patients experienced pain, and 12% reported unbearable pain. Twenty per cent of elderly care and general medical patients reported pain scores greater than or equal to 6. [2] In a survey of patients consecutively admitted to a London hospital, 13% had severe pain 15% had moderate pain at rest, and half had moderate or severe pain with movement. [3] A few more European surveys have also tried to assess the prevalence of pain among hospital patients. [4-6]

On a medical service the etiology of pain is diverse, and may be hard to ascertain. Data on the course and treatment of pain in medical inpatients are absent. Little is known about how intravenous opioid therapy, considered the treatment of choice for patients with severe, acute pain, is used on a medical service. In contrast to the post-operative setting, on a medical service the patient's course is less predictable, making it difficult to establish standards for when and how to change pain therapy and how to deliver it.

Textbooks and professional societies provide relatively straightforward guidance for managing acute pain in the perioperative setting and acute or chronic cancer pain. In contrast, in the U.S. no guidelines have not been proposed for the management of pain in acute inpatient medical care settings. Similarly, there are currently no performance measures in place to enhance pain management. The current VA Office of Research and Development pain-relevant research portfolio has no projects designed to examine the quality of pain care in the general medical or neurology ward setting.

HISTORICAL BACKGROUND

In 1986, the National Institutes of Health held a consensus development conference entitled "The Integrated Approach to the Management of Pain." [7] It focused on causes of undertreatment of pain, in particular, excessive concern about the problems of addiction and respiratory depression. The panel endorsed the principle that the most reliable measure of acute pain is the patient's self-report, but recognized limitations in the evidence, recommending future research on the "appropriateness of using existing research measures in clinical settings and…their validity as adjuncts to clinical judgments in pain assessment." They also cited innovations such as patient-controlled analgesia, but noted that clinical evaluation of PCA, sustained release formulations, epidural administration, and transdermal absorption of narcotic drugs to improve pain management were inadequate.

Since 1986, it has been widely recognized that a large minority of surgical patients have moderate to severe pain throughout their postoperative hospital course. [8] Poor pain management in inpatient surgical settings has been associated with slower recovery, [9] greater morbidity, longer lengths of stay, lower patient satisfaction, and higher costs of care, suggesting that optimal pain care in these settings is of utmost importance in promoting acute illness management, recovery, and adaptation.

In February, 1992, the Agency for Health Care Policy and Research released a guideline for the management of acute pain in trauma patients and in patients undergoing surgical or medical procedures. [10] In 1994, AHCPR published a guideline for managing cancer pain. [11] The AHCPR guidelines brought attention to deficiencies in the quality of care and endorsed several principles that became the foundation of inpatient pain management, including

- Clinicians should reassure patients and their families that most pain can be relieved safely and effectively.
- Clinicians should assess patients and, if pain is present, provide optimal relief throughout the course of illness.
- Health professionals should ask about pain, and the patient's self-report should be the primary source of assessment.
- Giving patients pain medicine only "as needed" resulted in prolonged delays because patients may delay asking for help.
- Aggressive prevention of pain is better than treatment because, once established, pain is more difficult to suppress.
- Physicians need to develop pain control plans before surgery and inform the patient what to expect in terms of pain during and after surgery.
- Fears of postsurgical addiction to opioids are generally groundless.
- Patient-controlled medication via infusion pumps is safe. [12]

The VHA National Pain Management Strategy, initiated November 12, 1998, established Pain Management as a national priority. The goals of the strategy included (1) the provision of a system-wide VHA standard of care for pain management to reduce suffering from preventable pain; (2) assurance that pain assessment is performed in a consistent manner and that pain treatment is prompt and appropriate; (3) the inclusion of patients and families as active participants in pain management; (4) the provision for continual monitoring and improvement in outcomes of pain treatment; (5) an interdisciplinary, multi-modal approach to pain management; and (6) assurance that clinicians practicing in the VA healthcare system are adequately prepared to assess and manage pain effectively. In 2000, VA published a toolkit for implementing these goals. (http://www1.va.gov/pain_management/docs/TOOLKIT.pdf)

The strategy led to rapid improvement in performance as measured by documentation of a pain assessment and pain care plans in the medical record and a lower proportion of patients with moderate or severe pain on study units. [13, 14] In 2000, for example, a survey conducted in VA inpatients with cancer found that only 42% of charts showed evidence that a pain rating scale was used [15] The VA and Institute for Healthcare Improvement initiated a collaborative project that used learning sessions, monthly team conference calls, and monitoring of results and sharing of improvement methods via Internet to promote routine assessment of pain and related goals. The learning sessions emphasized reliable and standardized measurement, strategies for interval sampling, and strategies for plotting and analyzing data. From May 2000 to January 2001, when the VA-IHI Joint Collaborative was conducted; moderate or severe pain on study units dropped from 24% to 17%; pain assessment increased from 75% to 85%; pain care plans for patients with at least mild pain increased from 58% to 78%; and number of patients provided with pain educational materials increased from 35% to 62%. [13, 14] By 2003, chart audit indicated that approximately 98% of veterans receiving care at a VHA facility had a documented pain score within the past 12 months. [16]

In July, 2002, VA/DoD developed a Clinical Practice Guideline for the management of acute post-operative pain. The basis for many of the recommendations was expert consensus rather than empirical evidence. To assess intensity, the VA/DOD CPG recommended use of a visual 1-10 numeric rating scale in the context of a complete pain history. Most of the guideline consists of site-specific recommendations for pharmacologic and nonpharmacologic therapy.

In 2003, VHA DIRECTIVE 2003-021 solidified previous accomplishments, leading to creation of a national pain management infrastructure. It requires implementation of "Pain as the 5th Vital Sign" in all clinical settings; establishment of pain management protocols in all clinical settings; and, for each patient, comprehensive pain assessment and development of a pain treatment plan.. It also encourages use of the pain reminders and dialogs sponsored by the VHA National Pain Management Strategy Coordinating Committee.

In 2004, the VHA National Pain Management Strategy Coordinating Committee issued a consensus statement on Assessing Pain in the Patient with Impaired Communication (available from http://www1.va.gov/Pain_Management/page.cfm?pg=41.)

METHODS

Topic Development

This project was nominated by Robert Kerns, Ph.D, VA National Coordinator for Pain Management, with input from a technical expert panel. Dr. Kerns proposed that we integrate the existing literature on the delivery of effective pain care in the acute inpatient medical ward. The results will be used to inform the VA's National Pain Management Strategy.

Key questions were discussed and finalized during a conference call that included the Steering Committee of the Evidence Synthesis Project and the Portland VAMC project site director. The questions apply only to the target population of inpatients on medical and neurology wards, not to surgical patients, patients with cancer, or patients with sickle cell crisis.

The final key questions are:

1. For inpatients who have acute pain, how do differences in timing and frequency of assessment, severity of pain, and follow-up of pain affect choice of treatment, clinical outcomes, and safety?

2. How do the timing and route of administration of pain interventions compare in effectiveness, adverse effects, and safety in these inpatient care settings?

3. For inpatients with impaired self-report due to any of several factors, including delirium or confusion, pre-existing severe dementia, closed head injury, stroke, and psychosis, how do differences in assessment and management of acute pain affect clinical outcomes or safety?

4. For inpatients with dependencies on tobacco, alcohol, stimulant, marijuana, or opioids, how do differences in assessment and management of acute pain affect clinical outcomes or safety? How do the assessment and management of acute pain differ between patients on prexisting opioid therapy and patients with opiate addiction?

We developed an analytic framework (Figure 1) to depict the clinical logic underlying these questions and the rationale for study selection. **Figure 1** shows the relationship between pain assessment and improved pain outcomes. For Key Question 1, we sought direct evidence linking improved pain assessment to improvements in pain outcomes (Arrow 1a), earlier or better treatment (Arrow 1b), or better detection and monitoring (Arrow 1c). Interventions to improve pain assessment could include a better choice of pain measure or different protocols for the frequency and timing of assessment.

Most interventions to improve pain assessment are part of broader systemwide programs that combine strategies to improve the timeliness and frequency of assessment with strategies to increase awareness and responsiveness to pain. When it comes to assessing effects on treatment and pain outcomes, the components aimed at assessment cannot be separated from other components, such as acute pain management teams. We discuss these interventions in the section about Key Question 2.

For Key Question 2, we assessed the timing and route of administration of therapy affect outcomes. At a system level, systemwide programs, acute pain management services, preprinted orders, clinical algorithms, and other management interventions may affect the timing and route of administration of pain treatments. At a more clinical level, we evaluated the use of intravenous versus other routes, prn orders, and patient-controlled analgesia.

Key Questions 3 and 4 follow the logic depicted in Figure 1, applied to patients with cognitive impairment and substance abuse problems, respectively.

Figure 1. Analytic Framework Showing Relationships among Key Questions.

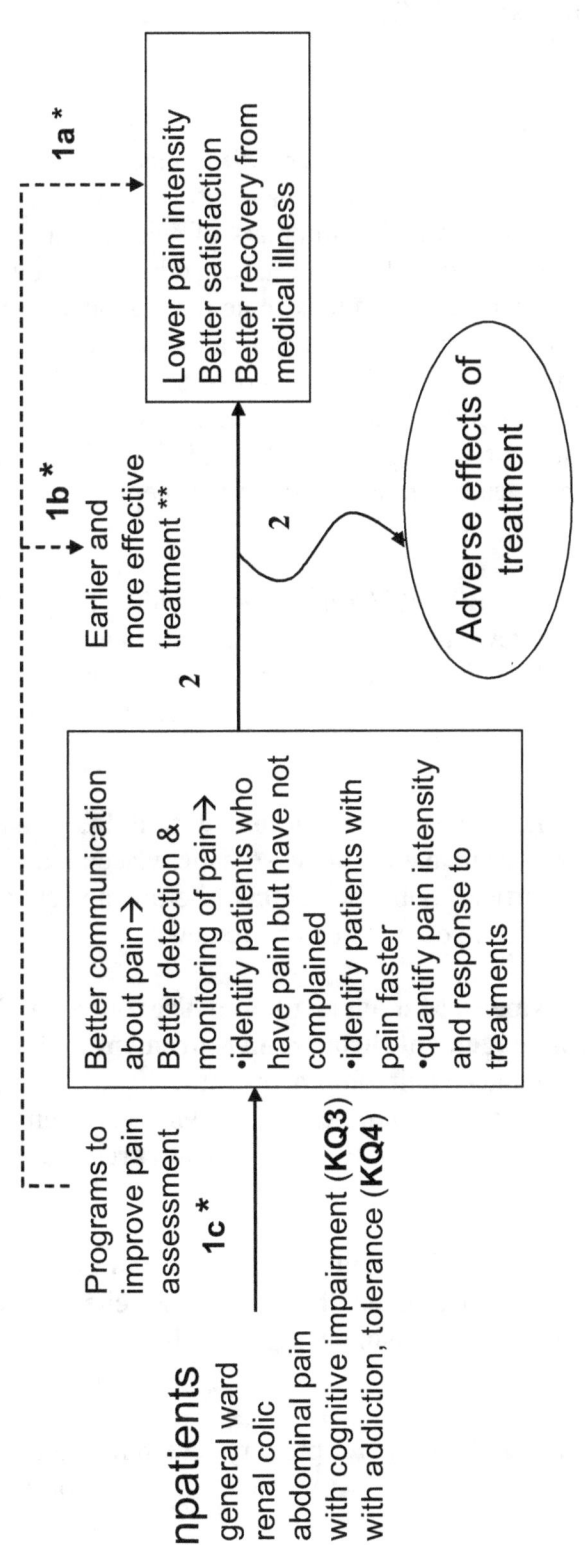

Inpatients
general ward
renal colic
abdominal pain
with cognitive impairment (**KQ3**)
with addiction, tolerance (**KQ4**)

Programs to improve pain assessment
1c *

Better communication about pain→
Better detection & monitoring of pain→
•identify patients who have pain but have not complained
•identify patients with pain faster
•quantify pain intensity and response to treatments

1b *
Earlier and more effective treatment **
2

1a *
Lower pain intensity
Better satisfaction
Better recovery from medical illness

2

Adverse effects of treatment

* KQ 1a, b, c The following types interventions might improve assessment:
• Better choice of pain measure
• Systemwide programs to improve the timeliness and frequency of assessment
• numerical pain assessment algorithms
• clinical pathways, guidelines, performance measurement

** KQ 2 Interventions include
• Acute pain management services and other system interventions
• Greater use of patient-controlled analgesia
• Greater use of IV vs. IM and PO routes
• Greater use of scheduled administration instead of just prn orders

VA-ESP April 2008

5

Search Strategy

Initially, we searched for previous systematic reviews in Medline, PubMed Clinical Queries, and the Cochrane Database of Systematic Reviews (1996 to April, 2007.) We identified several previous reviews:

Acute Pain Management: Scientific Evidence, 2nd edition (2005)[17]. The ANZCA review and guideline covers scientific articles published after 1998; it does not specify the closing date of the searches. ANZCA is a good-quality systematic review and guideline from Australia that provides the best available summary of research findings and recommendations for future research for many of the questions addressed in our report.[17] The guideline covers post-operative pain as well as acute pain associated with non-surgical conditions such as spinal cord injury, burns, cancer, acute zoster, neurological diseases, haematological disorders (e.g. sickle cell disease) and HIV/AIDS, as well as abdominal (e.g. renal and biliary colic), cardiac, musculoskeletal and orofacial pain and headache. It also covered acute pain management in the elderly, opioid-tolerant patients, patients with obstructive sleep apnea, renal or hepatic impairment or a substance abuse disorder.[18]

Institutional Approaches to Pain Assessment and Management (2003). This National Institute of Clinical Studies Literature Review, also from Australia, covers literature published between 1995 and May, 2002.[19] This systematic review covers multi-level institutional strategies, Acute Pain Services, and other dedicated-service strategies to improve pain assessment and management.

ICSI Healthcare Guideline: Assessment and Management of Acute Pain, 5th ed. 2006. This guideline provides algorithms for managing acute somatic, visceral, and neuropathic pain. It cites some pertinent articles published 2005 or before, and suggests some performance measures, [20] but is not based on a systematic review.

Pain: Current Understanding of Assessment, Management, and Treatments (2001) [21] and **Improving the quality of pain management through measurement and action (2003),**[22] address the application of continuous quality improvement techniques to pain assessment and management and the implementation of performance measurement processes. Both reports were prepared by the National Pharmaceutical Forum in collaboration with JCAHO.

International Association for the Study of Pain consensus guidelines on assessing pain in the elderly (2007) [23] While not evidence-based, these guidelines cite a large body of evidence about different approaches to assessing pain and includes a section about assessing pain in patients with cognitive impairment.

We proceeded to conduct a targeted search in Medline for primary research studies published from 1950 to July 2007 that address KQ1 or KQ2, the use of PCA for non-surgical pain. A list of studies included in the previous reviews, as well as the search terms and MeSH headings for the various search strategies, are found in Appendix A.

Study Selection

Two reviewers assessed for relevance the abstracts of citations identified from literature searches, using the criteria described in Appendix B. Full-text articles of potentially relevant abstracts were retrieved and a second review for inclusion was conducted by reapplying the inclusion criteria. Eligible articles had English-language abstracts and provided primary data relevant to the key questions. We included studies that were conducted in inpatients with acute pain and reported data on any of the following: Association between timing and frequency of pain assessment, severity of pain, and choice of treatment (e.g. regional blocks, medications, or other therapies); method of pain assessment (e.g. 11-point pain scale, visual analog scale, verbal descriptor scale; timing and route of administration of pain interventions (e.g. oral intermittent pharmacotherapy, intravenous therapy, psychological interventions, positioning, neural blockade, and patient-controlled analgesia); timeliness of enactment of treatment plans, changes in treatment plans; effect of coordination of care with the patient's primary care physician or with a pain consultation service on choice of treatment, clinical outcomes, and safety; patient outcomes, including degree of pain relief, pain intensity, emotional well-being, patient satisfaction, physical function, and fitness for rehabilitation of the underlying condition; safety outcomes; severity and frequency of side effects (including somnolence, respiratory depression, confusion, constipation, ileus, vomiting, non-allergic itching, weakness/numbness, and use of naloxone); length of stay; or follow-up of pain. We excluded studies of interventions that were not routinely available in the VA health system. We excluded studies of post-operative pain, sickle cell disease, cancer pain, chronic pain in patients hospitalized 10 days or longer for whom pain is chronic or refractory, except when studies of adverse effects were not available in the target population.

Data Abstraction and Quality Assessment

We abstracted the following data from included studies: Study Design/setting, Objective, eligibility criteria / method for assembling cohort, exclusion criteria, sample size, years of enrollment/observation, duration of follow-up, demographics, clinical category/baseline pain, method used to assess pain, intervention/exposure of interest, outcomes measured, potential confounders considered, results, conclusions. Although the studies were heterogeneous in design, objectives, and outcomes, we rated the quality of evidence of studies when applicable, using the criteria of the U.S. Preventive Services Task Force for evaluating randomized controlled trials and cohort and studies (Appendix C).[24]   For example, for randomized trials, we abstracted data on treatment allocation; \ the method of randomization; concealment of treatment allocation; similarity of groups at baseline regarding the most important prognostic indicators; blinding of the outcome assessor, care provider; and patients; loss to followup and use of intention-to-treat analysis.

Data Synthesis

We constructed evidence tables showing the study characteristics and results for all included studies, organized by key question, intervention, or clinical condition, as appropriate. We critically analyzed studies to compare their characteristics, methods, and findings. We compiled a summary of findings for each key question or clinical topic, and drew conclusions based on qualitative synthesis of the findings.

Rating the body of evidence

We assessed the overall quality of evidence for outcomes using a method developed by the Grade Working Group, which classified the grade of evidence across outcomes according to the following criteria:

o **High** = Further research is very unlikely to change our confidence on the estimate of effect.
o **Moderate** = Further research is likely to have an important impact on our confidence in the estimate of effect and may change the estimate.
o **Low** = Further research is very likely to have an important impact on our confidence in the estimate of effect and is likely to change the estimate.
o **Very Low** = Any estimate of effect is very uncertain.

GRADE also suggests using the following scheme for assigning the "grade" or strength of evidence:
Criteria for assigning grade of evidence
Type of evidence
Randomized trial = high
Observational study = low
Any other evidence = very low
Decrease grade if:
• Serious (-1) or very serious (-2) limitation to study quality
• Important inconsistency (-1)
• Some (-1) or major (-2) uncertainty about directness
• Imprecise or sparse data (-1)
• High probability of reporting bias (-1)
Increase grade if:
• Strong evidence of association-significant relative risk of > 2 (< 0.5) based on consistent evidence from two or more observational studies, with no plausible confounders (+1)
• Very strong evidence of association-significant relative risk of > 5 (< 0.2) based on direct evidence with no major threats to validity (+2)
• Evidence of a dose response gradient (+1)
• All plausible confounders would have reduced the effect (+1)

For this report, we used both this explicit scoring scheme and the global implicit judgment about "confidence" in the result.

Peer Review

Four peer reviewers provided feedback on the draft version of this report. Their comments and our responses are presented in Appendix D. One peer reviewer identified a potentially relevant article[25] and criticized the search strategy. In response, we conducted supplemental searches that identified 76 citations, two of which proved relevant to this report. The remaining citations concerned surgical, trauma, prehospital, emergency, and chronic patient settings.

RESULTS

There is much more evidence about outpatients with chronic pain, post-operative inpatients and patients with cancer than patients within the target population for this report. Throughout this report, we give precedence to the few studies that directly observed medical inpatients. We did not systematically review the literature about chronic pain, post-operative pain, or cancer pain assessment and management, but we invoke evidence from other populations when it is pertinent.

Key Question #1. How do differences in timing and frequency of assessment, severity of pain, and follow-up of pain affect choice of treatment, clinical outcomes, and safety?

Routine standardized pain assessment is usually implemented as part of a broader effort to coordinate pain management, particularly for post-operative patients. Usually, it is not possible to isolate timing and frequency of assessment from other components of these programs, which are discussed below in Key Question #2.

In medical inpatients with acute pain, does routine assessment of pain (for example, as the 5th vital sign) affect choice of treatment, clinical outcomes, and safety (Arrows 1a and 1b)?

We found no evidence that directly linked the timing, frequency, or choice of measure for assessment with the timeliness, choice, or safety of treatment specifically in medical inpatients. In the postoperative setting, routine numerical assessment of pain intensity increased utilization of intravenous analgesics and patient-controlled analgesia[26] and improved patient and staff satisfaction with pain management, but had unclear effects on pain severity and length of stay. In the emergency department, the addition of a mandated numeric pain scale to the medical record resulted in a significant increase in the proportion of patients in the ED who received analgesia, from 25% before implementation to 35% after implementation (Appendix E, Summary Table 1).[27] However, the extent of use on a medical ward of patient-controlled analgesia, regional analgesia, and specialized procedures is not well-documented, and experience in the postoperative and emergency care should not be generalized to this setting.

Does the choice of assessment measure affect choice of treatment, clinical outcomes, and safety?

As described above, since the 1980's there has been almost universal agreement that routine assessment of self-reported pain intensity is a better measure than pain assessed by a nurse or physician. This is because providers underestimate the severity of patients' pain in as many as half of cases. The disparity is greatest (60-68%) among patients with severe pain, and lowest (28-36%) among patients with mild pain.[28, 29] Routine assessment is encouraged because many patients, especially those who have cognitive impairment, do not always mention pain unless asked.

To be suitable for routine use as a vital sign, a self-reported pain assessment method must be simple to administer, easy for patients to understand, and responsive to changes in pain over time. Table 1 describes the most commonly used pain assessment measures. In case series, these measures have high internal consistency (Cronbach α 0.85 or greater) and at least fair test-retest reliability (r>0.5) in alert, cognitively intact individuals.[17, 23, 30] They are highly correlated with one another in such individuals, subject to patients' preferences for visual, numerical, or verbal descriptions and their willingness to use them. However, none of these assessment measures is intended to diagnose the cause of pain, and none are perfect across the entire spectrum of etiologies, pain types, comorbid conditions, and patient preferences encountered in a general medical ward.

The single dimension measures assess pain intensity. A 10-point verbal numeric rating scale (VRS or VNRS) is used widely within the VA health care system. Like all of these measures, the VRS has been evaluated more thoroughly in chronic pain and long-term care settings than in acute care settings, although there is one evaluation in medical inpatients undergoing common procedures.[31] That study compared a ten-point (N = 100) and five-point scale in 30 inpatients and found that the five-point scale exhibited better subject discrimination between experiences.

Table 1. Self-Assessment Pain Measures

Single Dimension	
Scale	**Description**
Visual analog scale	100 mm scale. Requires examiner to bring printed or on-screen scale and means for the patient to make a mark.
Verbal numeric rating scale	0 to 10 rating.
Verbal description scales	None-mild-moderate-severe.
Facial pain scales	Seven faces (0-6) or 10 faces (0-9) ranging from a neutral face (no pain) to a grimacing face (worst pain).
Multi Dimension	
Brief pain inventory	Assesses pain intensity and disability
McGill pain questionnaire	Assesses sensory, affective, and evaluative dimensions of pain

It is important to note the absence of evidence or consensus on what constitutes the *minimal clinically important difference* (MCID) for acute pain management in the hospital setting. The *minimal clinically important difference* is "…the smallest difference in score in the domain of interest which patients perceive as beneficial and which would mandate, in the absence of troublesome side effects and excessive cost, a change in the patient's management."[32] The MCID helps define a clinically significant response. A systematic review of pain intensity measurement found that the MCID was defined consistently across studies in chronic pain patients,[33] but this is not the case for acute nonsurgical pain. Determining the MCID for the VRS used in the VA system is a first step in studying and improving inpatient pain management.

Do protocols for assessing pain improve outcomes?

Many algorithms for assessing pain intensity and acting on the information are in use (for an example, see Figure 2.) Most algorithms directly link the intensity of pain to specific therapeutic actions, such as rapid administration of IV opioids.

We found no evaluations specifically of the effect of algorithms, preprinted orders, clinical pathways, or other protocols for assessing pain in the target population. In most cases, these algorithms are part of larger, institution-wide strategies to improve pain management. Although routine standardized assessment of self-reported pain severity is the cornerstone of these efforts, it is not possible to separate the effect of the assessment component from that of other components of these programs, such as an acute pain management service. The effect of these programs is addressed in Key Question #2.

With respect to safety, a study in cancer patients found that opioid-related oversedation and other adverse effects increased substantially after implementation of pain assessment on a numerical scale routinely with other vital signs.[34] This was the only study we identified that looked specifically at the association of routine use of numerical pain rating and adverse treatment effects. It was a retrospective review of records of patients who had experienced an adverse drug effect at the H. Lee Moffitt Cancer Center and Research Institute before (~1999) versus after (2002) implementation of a numerical pain treatment algorithm (Figure 3). Following implementation of the algorithm, there was a 2-fold increase in the risk of opioid oversedation (RR 2.22, 95% CI 1.07– 4.60), corresponding to an incidence from 11.0 per 100,000 inpatient hospital days to 24.5 per 100,000 inpatient hospital days post-NPTA (P < 0.001).

In the outpatient medical setting, VA has instituted several measures to improve pain management, including routine standardized assessment (or pain as the fifth vital sign), audit and feedback to clinical staff, specialist-level pain consultation services, nurse-level pain services, and palliative care services. A retrospective chart review study[35] and a prospective diagnostic test evaluation[36] cast doubt on the effectiveness of these interventions and on the accuracy of routine pain assessment, respectively, in the VA outpatient setting.

Assessment and Management of Pain in Inpatients

Figure 2. Inpatient Nursing Acute Pain Algorithm

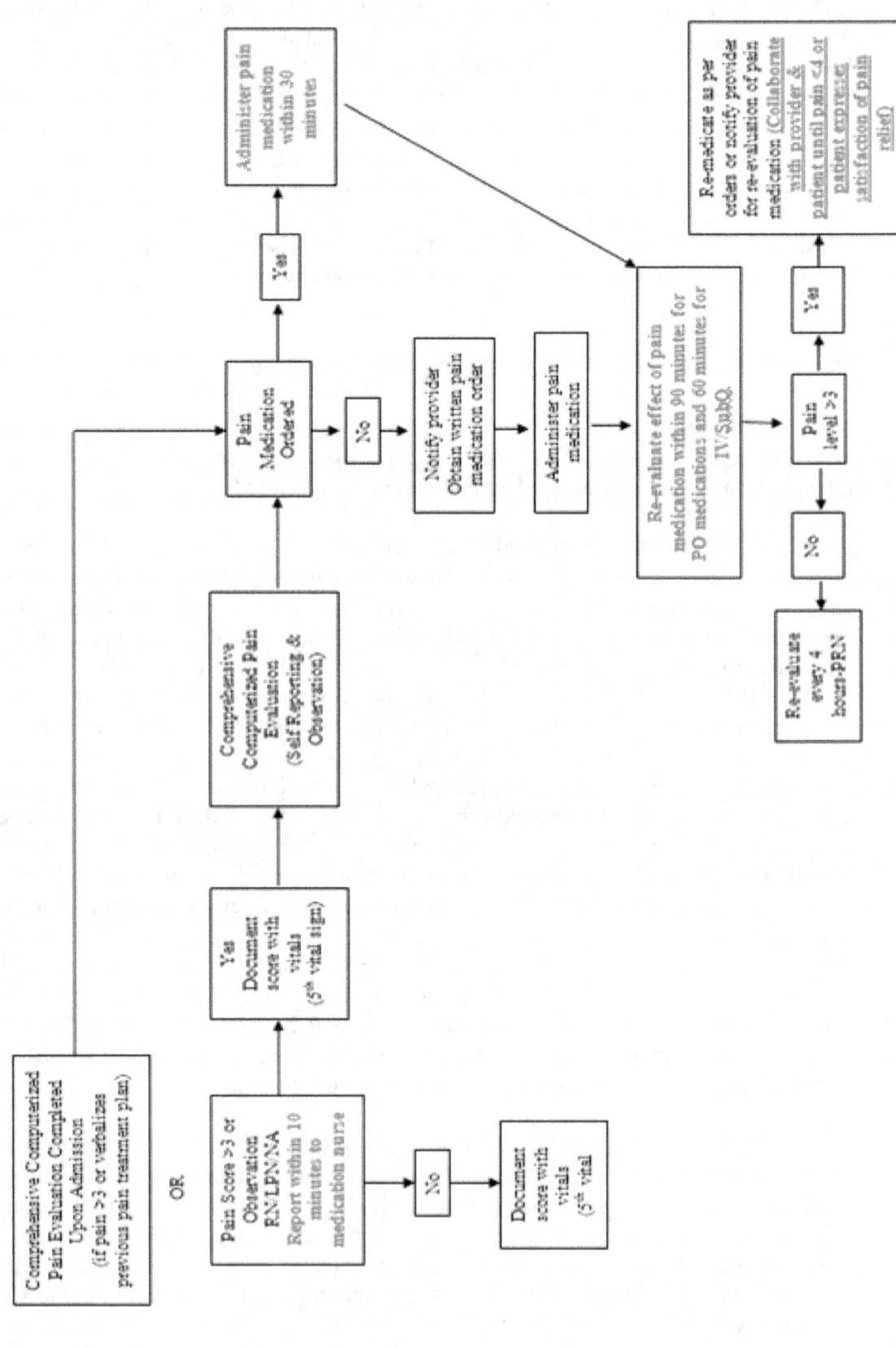

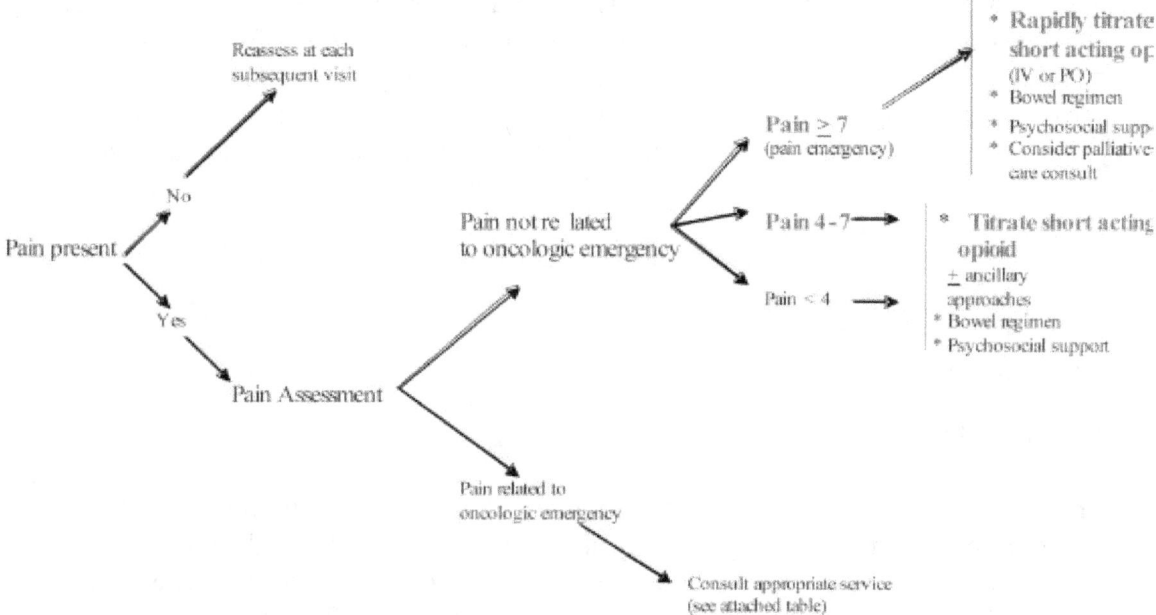

Figure 3. Pain Algorithm evaluated in Vila et al. [34]

Are there gaps in quality even when pain is assessed routinely?

We did not identify any studies of the timing or frequency of assessment of pain that focused on medical inpatients. However, evaluations conducted in the emergency room are relevant to medical inpatients, because patients headed for nonsurgical, noncancer wards are less likely to get adequate attention in the emergency room.

Surveys conducted in the late 1990's[37, 38] as well as more recent ones,[39] suggest that pain in emergency room patients is underdiagnosed and undertreated. . Potential risk factors for delayed or inadequate analgesia include female sex, less severe pain, and daytime admissions. Instituting routine assessment of pain, usually with an educational component, improved rates of assessment and treatment.[40, 41] In a University-based, single-institution, retrospective chart review study comparing outcomes in 521 medical encounters before and 479 after introduction of routine pain assessment of all patients in an emergency department, the addition of a mandated numeric pain scale increased the proportion of patients who received analgesia from 25% before implementation to 35% after implementation (p<0.001).[27] The time from triage to administration of analgesia improved on average from 152 to 113 minutes (but p>0.05). The standard triage form was revised to include a verbal numeric pain scale ranging from 0 to 10 in the vital signs section, and pain was measured at the same time as vital signs. The series included patients who presented with renal colic, extremity trauma, headache, ophthalmologic trauma or soft tissue injury (Appendix E, Summary Table 1).[27] A retrospective before-after study at a single hospital had similar results.[42]

Several chart review studies conducted in emergency departments focus on gaps in quality that remain even after institution of system changes. In the Nelson study just described, for example, patients with diagnostic uncertainty were less likely to receive analgesia compared with patients who received no workup (27% v. 34% respectively, p=0.0220). In a large, retrospective series from an Australian ED, patients who had a lower-priority triage score were nine times as likely as others to have a delay in treating pain; advanced age (>80 years) and admission to hospital were also associated with delays.[43] Documentation and treatment of pain deteriorates when the ED is busy (Appendix E, Summary Table 2).[44][45]

Specific Condition:

Abdominal Pain

Treating acute abdominal pain has traditionally been delayed until after evaluation by a surgeon, for concern that analgesia may alter the findings of physical examination, leading to misdiagnosis and management errors. A 1996 survey of 131 general surgeons in Iowa determined that 89% preferred to withhold analgesia for patients with acute abdomen until examined by a surgeon.[46]

In fact, there is good evidence that analgesia for acute abdomen is not only safe but beneficial because it facilitates more accurate diagnosis by localizing physical signs and allowing for more detailed examination by reducing patient stress.[47-49] More liberal use of analgesia has become common in practice. In a 2003 survey of ED physicians in 60 hospitals, 98.3% responded that it is the practice of their ED to administer narcotic analgesia to patients with acute abdomen prior to surgical consultation. Only 15.3% indicated that it is their practice to always verbally inform the surgeon prior to dosing the patient, and 49.2% reported the belief that analgesics aid in diagnostic accuracy.[50]

In a recent, good-quality systematic review and meta-analysis (Ranji et al), opioid administration had a negligible impact on clinical management and operative decision.[51] The review included 12 placebo-controlled RCTs of opioid analgesia in children and adults, reporting a total of 15 drug/dose comparisons. The combined findings of 11 comparisons from 9 studies in adults revealed a non-significant increase in changes in the physical examination with opioid administration, with a summary RR of 1.51 (95%CI 0.85 - 2.69). There was significant heterogeneity among the studies, and pain relief reported by the opioid group did not significantly differ from placebo in 3 of the comparisons. Most studies did not distinguish between potentially beneficial changes such as improved localization of tenderness and potentially harmful changes such as changes in peritoneal signs. Only 2 studies (including a study in children) specified that loss of peritoneal signs after analgesia occurred in 5.6% to 18.7% of patients with opioids, compared with 2.6% to 7.7% of those in the control group.

In an analysis of diagnostic accuracy in 4 adult studies, there was no significant change in the rate of incorrect management decisions with opioids compared with placebo (+0.3% absolute increase; 95%CI −4.1% to +4.7%). Analgesia was adequately greater than placebo in these studies, and no significant heterogeneity was found. The frequency of possible unnecessary surgeries was similar between opioid and control groups (7.6% v 7.9%). Meta-analysis showed non-significantly fewer unnecessary surgeries among patients with opioids. The reviewers concluded that opioid administration appears to have negligible impact on clinical management, in that 909 patients would need to receive opioids to result in 1 potential management error.[51] A trial intravenous morphine vs. placebo, published too recently to be included in the Ranji review, supported these findings.[52]

Waiting for a surgical consultant is only one cause of delay in treating abdominal pain. One systematic review[51] and one primary study[53] examined the timing of assessment and analgesia for acute abdominal pain. Three studies examined the relation of severity of pain, ED crowding, and other factors to timing of assessment and treatment (Appendix E, Summary Table 2).[39, 43, 44] Immediate referral to surgery when the patient with acute abdominal pain comes to the ED reduces, but does not eliminate, delay in analgesia. A 2004 study in such a setting examined the factors associated with waiting time from prescription to administration of analgesia among 100 consecutive patients presenting with acute abdomen at a hospital in the UK.[53] Despite having direct access to an on-call surgical service, thus eliminating the referral delay and the need to withhold analgesia in the interim, the administration of analgesia to patients in this setting was heterogeneous. Sixty-seven percent of patients received analgesia within 1 hour, and 22% waited 2-14 hours after presentation. The study found that severe pain was more likely to be treated quickly, that females had a longer mean wait time than males (129 min v. 69 min, p=0.09), and patients admitted at night waited less time (mean 76 min) than those during the day (mean 114 min). The timing of analgesia was not associated with clinical diagnosis or patient age. Diclofenac was the most commonly prescribed analgesic (37%), followed by pethidine (26%). No patients received analgesia intravenously, and 80% received analgesia through the intramuscular route. Nearly a fourth of patients reported that the analgesia received was inadequate.

Key Question #2. How do the timing and route of administration of pain interventions compare in effectiveness, adverse effects, and safety in inpatient care settings?

In general, pain in medical inpatients is managed by the primary team, with involvement from an acute pain team on a consultation basis. There are no programs directed mainly at improving pain management in medical inpatients who do not have cancer and are not suffering from a terminal disease. For clinicians, one of the main clinical management questions is when to use pain and palliative care consultants for such patients, and whether they improve outcomes in this setting. Another important question is whether use of PCA and other modalities improve control of pain and satisfaction of patients and staff.

Do acute pain management teams and other institutional initiatives improve effectiveness, adverse effects, and safety in medical inpatients?

Most institution-wide efforts to improve pain assessment and management aim to influence the timing and route of administration of pain interventions. As mentioned earlier, it is usually not possible to isolate the effect of administration of treatments from other elements of multifaceted programs. However, it is worth examining the overall effects of these programs and their effect on how treatments are administered.

Table 2. Some elements of institution-wide efforts to improve pain assessment and management.

Identify key opinion leaders from relevant disciplines to form a steering committee.
Identify pain assessment problems.
Critically evaluate the applicability of guidelines and other scientific literature on pain assessment to a particular setting.
Form continuous quality improvement team to map, monitor, and evaluate care processes.
Develop and implement pain management standards.
Develop critical pathways, preprinted or prespecified electronic orders, paper or electronic pain assessment and management algorithms.
Staff education "pain management toolbox" (printed materials, videotapes, weekly "pain rounds", invited lectures)
Form an acute pain management consultation service.
Monitoring to determine whether pain treatments have been effective (Pain as a fifth vital sign.)
Chart audit, surveys of patient satisfaction.

Elements of institution-wide interventions vary, but most incorporate a majority of the elements listed in Table 2. [19] For example, the VHA/Institute for Healthcare Improvement (IHI) Pain Management Collaborative, employed system-wide strategies to modify existing pain assessment and management practices within the VHA.[16] Seventy teams from 22 VISNs throughout the U.S. participated in the 6-month joint Collaborative, with the following measurable objectives: to reduce the prevalence of severe pain by 25%; increase assessment such that 100% of patients will have their pain assessed; increase by 20% the documentation of plan of care among patients with a pain score >=4; and to provide appropriate pain management education to at least 50% of patients with a pain score of >=4. The strategic goals included: 1) provision of a system-wide VHA standard of care for pain management; 2) assurance that pain assessment is performed in a consistent manner and that pain treatment is prompt and appropriate; 3) the inclusion of patients and families as active participants in pain management; 4) continual monitoring and improvement in outcomes of pain treatment; 5) an interdisciplinary, multi-modal approach to pain management; and 6) assurance that clinicians practicing in the VA health care system are adequately prepared to assess and manage pain effectively.

The VHA/IHI Collaborative used learning sessions, monthly team conference calls, and monitoring of results and sharing of improvement methods via Internet. The learning sessions emphasized reliable and standardized measurement, strategies for interval sampling, and strategies for plotting and analyzing data. Data collection methods were specific to each clinical setting: for inpatients and long-term care settings, at least 2 patients each day were selected randomly; for Emergency Departments, teams could either select time points (e.g. 10AM and 3PM) or to select 2 charts randomly each data for data abstraction; for ambulatory settings, medical records of patients who visited during the month were sampled, excluding patients who were being seen for the first time in primary care. The project did not include a concurrent control group. Three of the 4 objectives were met, and most of the improvements occurred during the first 3 months of the collaboration, and sustained during the next 3 months. The goal of 100% patient assessment was not met, although the frequency of pain assessment increased from 58% to 85% of patients during the collaboration period.

Most primary studies in this review focused on postoperative or cancer pain, and were uncontrolled (see next section.) We identified one controlled trial, published since this review, which included medical inpatients. It found that a multifaceted intervention improved assessment of pain, but did not affect pain intensity or duration.[54] The trial enrolled a random sample of 3964 English-speaking, cognitively intact subjects admitted to matched medical/surgical units (3 general medicine, 2 general surgery, 2 specialty surgery, 1 oncology, and 1 mixed oncology/general medicine) at Mount Sinai Hospital in New York. Usual care required that pain be assessed at least once per shift using a 4-point scale. The intervention included, in phases: education, standardized pain assessment using a 1- or 4-item (enhanced) pain scale, audit and feedback of pain scores to nursing staff, and a computerized decision support system to guide analgesic prescribing. The enhanced pain assessment asked patients to rate current pain, worst pain, pain relief, and whether the level of pain was acceptable on 4-pt scales. Patients were interviewed within 48 hrs of admission and then once daily. An enhanced pain assessment that asked inpatients to rate current pain, worst pain, pain relief, and whether the pain level was acceptable on 4-point scales increased the likelihood of pain assessment, improved documentation of pain, and resulted in increased analgesia prescribing.[54] The percentage of patients who received at least 1 pain assessment per day increased from 32.1% with the standard pain assessment to 79.3% when the enhanced pain scale was combined with the CSS, and to >80% when combined with audit and feedback.

Although the enhanced pain scale and other interventions improved pain assessment and increased analgesic prescribing, the intervention did not alter severity of pain. The percentage of patients who had 72-96 hours of persistent pain following study enrollment and overall mean pain scores remained relatively constant across both blocks and all phases of the study.

Do acute pain management teams and other institutional initiatives improve effectiveness, adverse effects, and safety in other settings?

In patients with cancer, most programs include one or more of the following components: professional and patient education, instituting regular pain assessment (pain as a vital sign), audit of pain results and feedback to clinical staff, computerized decisional support systems, and specialist-level pain consultation services.[55] Techniques for improving assessment and documentation of cancer pain included graphic recording on bedside charts, standardized pain assessment flow sheets, incorporation of both formal education and assessment tools, and institution-wide multidisciplinary programs. A 2007 systematic review identified 10 studies of these interventions; several of them included at least some medical inpatients who did not have cancer. These studies demonstrated that routine pain assessment improved patient and staff satisfaction with pain management and improved documentation, but did not improve overall pain scores or pain severity. [55]

There is much more evidence from the post-operative setting. A 2003 systematic review on institutional approaches to pain assessment and management, conducted in Australia by the Department of Public Health and the National Institute of Clinical Studies (NICS) identified 3 comparative studies and 29 before-and-after studies of the effect of institutional pain management programs on treatment and patient outcomes.[19] Most of these programs implemented routine numerical pain assessment and some form of a pain management team. Overall, interventions improve pain assessment indicators such as use of pain intensity scales, pain flow sheets, a pain plan of care, and documentation of location and quality of pain, and response to treatment. Interventions also increase administration of scheduled (rather than prn) pain medication, reduce use of the IM route, and increase the use of intravenous analgesia and of PCA.

While pain management teams and other system interventions improved the timeliness and frequency of pain assessment, evidence for improvements in pain outcomes was conflicting. The NICS review included 10 studies on dedicated service strategies.[19] These included 9 studies on the introduction of pain management teams, most commonly an Acute Pain Service, and 1 before-and-after study of the introduction of a pain monitoring specialist. Two studies were multi-center studies that compared an intervention group with a control group where standard patient care was maintained (i.e. did not introduce a dedicated pain management service).

The results of the controlled studies suggest that Acute Pain Services in tertiary settings reduce the intensity of pain experienced by patients and improve their functional ability, although these effects were not always determined to be clinically important. The use of a dedicated service strategy increased use of patient-controlled analgesia and IV opioids, while IM administration decreased substantially. Prescribing practices also appeared to be altered in that NSAID and paracetamol use increased significantly. A statistically and clinically important improvement in patient satisfaction with pain management was also observed. Analgesia-related adverse effects, such as nausea, vomiting, sedation, diarrhea, and hypotension, appear to be reduced after the introduction of a dedicated service strategy.

The review also examined multi-level strategies, in which strategies were developed to modify existing pain assessment and management policies, procedures, and practices at all levels of the institution. Most multi-level strategies included staff education and the use of standardized pain assessment methods. The integration of pain assessment as a "5th vital sign" was included in two studies. The effects of multi-level strategies on pain reduction, functional ability, and patient satisfaction were variable. Only one study of a multi-level strategy used a control group. The body of evidence on institutional approaches to pain assessment and management was of limited quality overall.[19]

In summary, institutional interventions improved pain assessment and documentation and staff awareness of pain, and increased use of analgesics. There was only poor-quality evidence that these programs improved safety. Most importantly, the programs' effect on patient levels of pain was inconsistent; in the relatively higher-quality studies, programs did not improve pain.

How does coordination with the patient's primary care physician affect outcomes?

We found no evidence about the value of coordinating care with the patient's primary care physician.

How does the choice of treatment modality affect effectiveness, adverse effects, and safety in inpatient care settings?

Treatment options for pain management are listed in Table 3 below.[1, 17, 20] There is a glaring lack of comparative studies of different agents and methods of administration in the general inpatient setting.

Table 3. Treatments for acute pain

TREATMENTS	COMMENTS

Psychological and physical methods
    Providing information
    Relaxation
    Attentional techniques
    Hypnosis
    Cognitive-behavioral interventions
    TENS
    Acupuncture
    Positioning
    Manual and massage therapies
    Heat and cold
	--- 	

TREATMENTS	COMMENTS
Non-steroidal anti-inflammatory drugs, acetaminophen, topical therapies, combinations	Bleeding, renal, coagulation problems and fluid retention (NSAIDs)
Nitrous oxide, corticosteroids, ketamine, clonidine	Role in inpatient medical patients unclear.

Opioids
 	
   Delivery methods
   oral intermittent
   subcutaneous
   transdermal
   IM
   IV administered by a nurse on request
   IV administered by a nurse on a schedule
   Patient-controlled analgesia
 	
   Adjuvant drugs
   Antiemetics
   Ketamine
   Naloxone
   Clonidine
	First-line treatment for severe, acute pain.
	
	No clear evidence that any opioid is better in medical inpatients.
	
	Requires good staffing levels to minimize delay between need and injection (or between need and setting up PCA)
	
	Risks of PCA vs. other methods of administration are similar in surgical patients but have not been studied in medical inpatients.
	
	Respiratory depression, diminished level of consciousness, constipation, urinary retention, and other complications are common side effects.

Regional Analgesia
 	
   Neuraxial blockade
   Peripheral,n. blockades
   Paravertebral, intercostal, interpleural, etc
	Role in inpatient medical patients unclear.

Epidural Analgesia
   Thoracic or Lumbar
   Usually opioid+local anesthetic and sometimes epinephrine
   Sometimes patient-controlled
	Role in inpatient medical patients unclear.
	
	The risks are those of an epidural (neurological damage, epidural hematoma, epidural abscess)l +those of the drugs (local anesthetic+opioid)

Specialized procedures (eg, joint injection, wound infiltration)	
SYSTEM INTERVENTIONS	
Use of acute pain management team	
Coordination of care with primary care physician	

Effectiveness and safety of patient-controlled analgesia (PCA)

PCA refers to methods of pain relief that allow a patient to self-administer small doses of an analgesic agent as required. The concept of PCA was introduced in 1970, but the method did not become popular until the 1980's, when improvements in infusion pump technology made wider use of PCA in post-operative patients feasible. [56]

The vast majority of studies on the use of PCA pertained to postoperative pain or acute pain due to exacerbation of chronic medical conditions such as sickle cell crisis or cancer. PCA has also been evaluated in patients with fractures or other traumatic injury (see Appendix E, Summary Table 3).[57-60]

Early trials of PCA compared it with intermittent, intramuscular opioid injections administered by a nurse. More recent trials compare PCA to epidural analgesia. All of these trials were conducted in the setting of post-anesthesia care units or, subsequently, a (postoperative) surgical ward.

In post-operative patients, regional and epidural analgesia have been compared with intravenous opioids, administered intermittently or by patient-controlled analgesia (PCA). Recent systematic reviews identified surgical conditions in which regional analgesia provides superior pain relief compared with opioids, but could not confirm or deny a relationship between the choice of postoperative analgesic techniques on major mortality or morbidity.[61, 62] Other systematic reviews have found that, after surgery, patients using PCA consumed higher amounts of opioids and had better pain control and higher satisfaction than patients treated with prn or scheduled opioid treatments, with no higher incidence of most side effects [63-65] Comparative evidence is generally favorable to regional analgesia for certain surgeries, but overall evidence comparing continuous epidural analgesia and PCA is not conclusive. [66-70]

The evidence summarized in these reviews has low applicability to medical inpatients, where the course of pain as well as staffing and monitoring procedures differ from those of the post-anesthesia unit. There is almost no information on the use or safety of PCA in a medical ward setting. A fair-quality, non-blinded RCT compared the effectiveness of morphine delivered by nurses as needed versus by IV-PCA in 86 patients who presented to the ED with a pain score of 7+ due to traumatic injury, most commonly fracture (74% in the PCA group, 53.4% of controls), and found that pain relief and patient satisfaction were similar between the treatment modalities.[58] Pain scores and physiological measurements were collected at 0, 5, 15, 30, 45, 60, 90, and 120 minutes. Although the PCA group used more than twice as much morphine than controls (mean total 18.83 mg vs. 7.65; mean usage rate 7.26 mg/h v. 4.03 mg/h), the mean VAS pain scores were the same (4.8) in treatment both groups, and there were no significant differences between groups in the satisfaction questionnaires. An area-under-the-curve analysis of VAS scores confirmed no significant difference between groups. The investigators noted the limitation that nurse behavior might have been influenced by the presence of researchers to optimize delivery of pain relief, given the non-blinded design of the study.

Most of the evidence on the adverse effects of PCA was derived from the experience of patients with postoperative pain or chronic conditions.[17, 71-73] The opioid-related side effects from IV PCA are the same as those for intermittent opioid analgesic regimens, and include respiratory depression, sedation, constipation, pruritis, nausea, and vomiting. Patient factors and misuse of the PCA device by family members, however, may lead to the inappropriate use of PCA,[71] and cases of oversedation caused by equipment programming mishaps have been reported.[73]

In patients with acute thoracic pain from traumatic injury, analgesia with IV-morphine PCA was equivalent to morphine administered PRN in one study[58] and to nebulized morphine in another study,[57] but inferior to epidural analgesia in 2 studies.[59, 60] Most patients in these studies had suffered fractures, though the populations varied in the type and severity of the injuries.

The lack of data on the use and safety of PCA in medical patients is concerning, for there are protocols for post-op management but not for medical patients. Pain improves predictably in the post-operative period, making weaning protocols easier to implement. Also, use of PCA is integrated into staff routines and monitoring protocols. None of these characteristics apply to medical inpatients.

Specific Conditions

Renal colic and biliary stone pain

Most evidence about treating renal colic is old and addresses whether to use IM, SC, or IV analgesics. The main findings, discussed in more detail below, are (1) NSAIDs provide effective analgesia for acute renal colic, and act more quickly through the IV route than by IM or PR 2) Opioids provide analgesia that is equivalent to NSAIDs but result in a higher incidence of vomiting and other adverse events, particularly pethidine 3) Hydromorphone provided superior pain relief and led to fewer hospital admissions compared with meperidine in one study. 4) Intramuscular injection of opioids should not be used because it causes more discomfort and complications than subcutaneous injection and relieves pain no faster. Many studies excluded patients who had negative followup investigations for biliary stone or renal calculi, which may limit the applicability of findings to all patients presenting with pain from these suspected causes (see Appendix E, Summary Table 4).

A 1998 systematic review of NSAIDS included 3 trials in renal colic in which the same drug was compared by different routes.[74] Two trials compared 50 mg intravenous vs. 100 mg rectal indomethacin.[75, 76] The 3rd trial compared IV with IM administration of dipyrone and diclofenac in 6 comparisons: dipyrone 1g or 2g IM + placebo IV; dipyrone 1g or 2g IV + placebo IM; diclofenac 75 mg IM + placebo IV; diclofenac 75 mg IV + placebo IM.[77] In all 3 trials, the NSAID acted more quickly through the intravenous route than rectal or intramuscular. The difference was significant, but evident only during the first 10 to 20 minutes.

A 2007 Cochrane review of NSAIDS vs. opioids for acute renal colic found that both NSAIDs and opioids provide effective analgesia in acute renal colic, but opioids, particularly pethidine, result in a higher incidence of vomiting and other adverse events.[78] Five different NSAIDS (diclofenac, indomethacin, indoprofen, ketorolac, tenoxicam) and 7 opioids were studied in 20 trials from 9 countries with a total of 1613 participants.[78] The intramuscular route was most commonly used for each drug type (10 trials), followed by the intravenous route (7 trials). Patients receiving NSAIDs reported lower pain scores than patients receiving opioids in 10 of 13 studies, though the differences were small. Pooled results on efficacy were not available due to heterogeneity between studies. Patients treated with NSAIDs were significantly less likely to require rescue analgesia (RR 0.75, 95%CI 0.61-0.93). A higher incidence of adverse events occurred with opioids than with NSAIDs in the majority of trials, and pethidine in particular was associated with a higher rate of vomiting. Most studies included only participants with renal calculi confirrmed on subsequent testing and excluded patients with negative results on followup tests. These exclusions may limit the applicability of findings to all patients who present with the clinical picture of renal colic.

A 2007 Cochrane review of hydromorphone in acute and chronic pain[79] identified one trial in patients with renal colic,[80] and one trial in patients with biliary stone pain.[81] In a fair-quality double-blind RCT, patients with renal colic were randomized to receive either 50 mg meperidine or 1 mg hydromorphone IV, and their pain scores were measured on a 10-cm VAS were recorded at t=0, 15, 30, 60, and 120 minutes.[80] Patients who received hydromorphone achieved more pain relief, required less rescue medication, underwent fewer IV pyelograms, and avoided hospital admission more frequently than did patients who received meperedine. A poor-quality unblinded trial in 42 patients with biliary stone pain compared subcutaneous injection of 1mL dihydromporphinone with 50 mg indomethacin IV.[81] Eight initially enrolled patients were excluded from analysis because follow-up X-ray or ultrasonogram investigations were negative for these patients. Pain was evaluated by VAS at baseline and at 10 and 30 minutes after drug injection. Indomethacin and dihydromorphinone were equally effective at reducing pain in patients with acute attacks of biliary stone pain. VAS scores at 0, 10, and 30 minutes were 71.8, 44.1, and 14.2 in the dihydromorphinone group, compared with 68.5, 32.4, 15.8 in the indomethacin group, and the differences between groups were not statistically significant. No serious side effects were observed with either drug. The lack of patient blinding was a limitation in this study, and the exclusion of patients who were later found to be negative for biliary stone may limit applicability of findings to all patients who present with biliary stone pain.

Phantom Limb Pain

Phantom limb pain is a form of neuropathic pain perceived in the missing limb after amputation that is distinct from pain in the residual portion of the limb or stump, and other non-painful sensation of the missing limb. In trials of perioperative interventions, the prevalence of phantom limb pain after amputation among control subjects ranged from 56-82% at day 7, 39-73% at 6 months, and 27-78% at 12 months.[82] A survey in 1980 identified more than 50 different therapies in use for the treatment of phantom limb pain [83], suggesting limited consensus on the effectiveness of treatment.

A good-quality systematic review sought to determine the optimal management of acute and chronic phantom limb pain, and identified 12 controlled trials that reported phantom pain as an outcome (see Appendix E, Summary Table 5).[82] The included studies were published between 1985-1997, and the 12 trials included a combined total of 375 male and female patients, ages 47-75. Trials were included if they involved a control group and examined any intervention for PLP, regardless of methodology. Interventions involving treatments before and during the amputation were included, as well as treatments for chronic pain.

Trials were divided into 2 groups based on the timing of intervention (early vs. late): 8 trials of preoperative, intraoperative, and early postoperative interventions at <2 weeks, and 4 trials of late (>2 weeks) postoperative interventions. Among the 8 early intervention trials, 3 used epidural anesthesia, 3 used regional nerve blocks, 1 used intravenous calcitonin, and 1 used transcutaneous electrical nerve stimulation (TENS). Controls in these studies received a placebo consisting of a saline infusion or epidural anesthesia consisting of on-demand opioid analgesia. The 4 trials of late postoperative interventions studied the use of TENS, a crossover study comparing the use of a metal threaded sock (Farabloc) vs. no treatment, vibratory stimulation vs. placebo stimulation, and intravenously infused ketamine vs. saline. Subjects served as their own controls in these studies, and in most of the early treatment studies the control group received active treatment with opioid analgesics. No trials examined commonly recommended oral drugs, such as membrane stabilizers or tricyclic antidepressants.

Among the 8 early intervention trials, 3 trials of preoperative epidural pain relief reported mixed results. Three other trials assessed sciatic or posterior tibial nerve blocks with perineural and intraneural bupivacaine blocks during or immediately after surgery, and found no differences in pain between the intervention and control groups in the postacute period, measured at various timepoints up to 12 months after surgery. In a trial of calcium calcitonin (200 IU) and a trial of early TENS, reduced phantom limb pain was observed in the early postoperative period but not in longer-term followup. In trials of the late postoperative phase, Farabloc, low-frequency TENS applied to the ear, and ketamine provided a modest short-term reduction in phantom limb pain and paresthesia. Another late-treatment trial examined TENS at the site of pain but findings were inconclusive. Several studies were limited by small sample sizes, and high loss rates from dropouts, re-amputations, and mortality.

The review[82] concluded that there is little evidence from randomized trials to support any particular treatment of phantom limb pain either in the acute perioperative period or later. Evidence on preemptive epidurals, early regional nerve blocks, and mechanical vibratory stimulation provides inconsistent support for these treatments.

Studies of the effectiveness of other treatments for phantom limb pain were identified in the ANZCA report.[17] Early postoperative infusion salmon calcitonin was effective at reducing phantom limb pain compared with placebo, in a double-blind crossover trial (n=21). One week after the first treatment, 90% of patients had pain relief of more than

50%, 76% were completely pain free, and 71% never experienced phantom limb pain again. One year later, 8 (62%) of the 13 surviving patients still had more than 75% phantom limb pain relief.[84] In single studies, ketamine,[85] oral slow-release morphine,[86] IV infusion of morphine,[87] and gabapentin[88] were also effective in reducing phantom limb pain. Lidocaine had no effect on phantom limb pain, but significantly reduced stump pain in one study.[87]

The ANZCA report also identified three studies of interventions to prevent phantom limb pain.[17] A small observational study found that in 14 patients given a bolus dose of ketamine followed by an infusion, begun preoperatively and continued for 72 hours postoperatively, the incidence of severe phantom limb pain was reduced, compared with no ketamine in 14 historical controls.[89] An RCT that compared perioperative intravenous ketamine infusion to saline infusion in 45 patients found the incidence of phantom limb pain at 6 months post-amputation was lower in the ketamine group than the control group (47% v. 71%) but the difference was not statistically significant.[90] A review of the efficacy of perioperative epidural analgesia determined that the incidence of severe of phantom limb pain was reduced though not completely abolished 12 months after amputation (NNT = 5.8, 95% CI 3.2-28.6).[91] A non-pharmacological treatment for phantom limb pain was effective in a study of sensory discrimination training.[92]

Overall there is a paucity of evidence to guide specific specific treatment of phantom limb pain. Single studies showed evidence of the effectiveness of various therapies (calcitonin, morphine, ketamine, gabapentin, and sensory discrimination training), and perioperative studies of ketamine and epidural analgesia showed reduced incidence of phantom limb pain, but these studies were limited by small sample size.

Key Question #3. For inpatients with impaired self-report due to any of several factors, including delirium or confusion, pre-existing severe dementia, closed head injury, stroke, and psychosis, how do differences in assessment and management of acute pain affect clinical outcomes or safety?

Cognitive impairment complicates assessment and treatment of pain. Several studies have reported underestimation by providers of pain in cognitively impaired patients.[93] Most studies of pain in cognitively impaired individuals were conducted in nursing homes,[94] where chronic dementia is the most prevalent cause of cognitive impairment. A large bibliography of articles, guidelines, and quality indicators for pain management in nursing homes is available at http://medqic.org/

Briefly, most guidelines for the management of pain in patients with cognitive impairment emphasize principles set forth in a 1993 article by Parmelee[95] and modified by others[96-98]:

1. Assess all patients for cognitive impairment using a Mini-Mental State Examination (MMSE).

2. Mildly impaired individuals are almost as able as cognitively intact individuals to accurately report their pain.
3. Impaired patients with communication skills will not neglect reporting of pain when queried specifically.
4. In moderately and severely impaired individuals, try several different scales. Most moderately and severely impaired individuals can understand at least one pain assessment scale (verbal, horizontal visual, or faces)[99,100]
5. Self-report can also be improved by other strategies, such as asking the patient to describe painful events that have been experienced that correspond to different pain intensities. Patients can be prompted by asking about common events that occur in a clinical setting such as needle sticks. [98]
6. Markedly impaired patients report less intense pain and a smaller number of pain complaints than the mildly impaired.
7. For patients who are impaired and deny pain or do not respond to questions about pain, use an observational assessment tool to screen for pain.

This guidance, intended for use in nursing homes, has limited applicability to the medical inpatient setting, where delirium is a much more common cause of cognitive impairment. Buffum reviewed the sparse literature on assessing and managing pain in delirious patients and identified a long list of research gaps and priorities.[97] Except for some surveys of the prevalence of delirium among inpatients (cited in Buffum), we identified no relevant studies of pain assessment or management in patients with delirium.

Most studies of pain and cognitive impairment focus on assessment. There is fair evidence from one prospective cohort study[99] that most cognitively impaired individuals can understand at least one self-assessment measure. This study was conducted in a series of 160 consecutive inpatients, recruited from 2 Swiss hospitals and referred for dementia consultation. The investigators administered 4 self-assessment scales (horizontal VAS, vertical VAS, faces pain scale, verbal rating scale) and one observational rating scale (the Doloplus scale, developed to assess pain in older people with communicative disorders).[99] Patients were considered to have understood a scale if on both self-assessments the patient was able to explain it use and could correctly indicate which position on the scale corresponded to no pain at all, and which position corresponded to the most severe pain. Comprehension of at least 1 scale was demonstrated by 40% of patients with severe dementia, 90% of patients with moderate dementia, and 97% of patients with mild dementia. The correlation between the self-assessment scales was high (Spearman's r_s = 0.81-0.95, $p<0.001$). The Doloplus observational rating scale correlated only moderately with self-assessment by the patient (Spearman's r_s = 0.31-0.40, $p<0.05$), and the strength of the correlations did not increase in patients with moderate to severe pain. The investigators in this study concluded that the majority of hospitalized patients with dementia can reliably use self-assessment pain scales, and that observational scales tend to underestimate pain intensity and should be reserved for patients who have demonstrated that they cannot complete a self-assessment. One limitation of this study is that none of the severely demented patients who could demonstrate appropriate use of the self-assessment scales reported experiencing any pain. This means that, at best, the authors' conclusions about the usefulness of the self-assessment scales may apply only to distinguishing between some pain and none—that is, the study provides no evidence about the scaling properties of self-assessment scales in severely demented patients.

Another study compared the psychometric properties of 4 established pain scales between moderately impaired (MMSE 13-21, n=42) and cognitively unimpaired (MMSE 22-30, n=33) hospitalized older adults (mean age 76 yrs) with pain at admission.[101] Patients participated in the study for 14 days. On days 1-7, participants were visited 3 times per day and asked to rate their current pain on each of 4 scales: 1) a 5-pt verbal rating scale; 2) a 7-pt faces scale; 3) a horizontal 21-point box scale; 4) 2 vertical 21-point box scales. Patients were also asked to make retrospective ratings at the end of the day and at weekly time points, with reference to usual, worst, and least pain levels, using each of the 4 scales for each rating. The study sought to determine the effect of mental status on pain rating; scale redundancy, scale reliability, validity/current pain bias (whether a retrospective pain rating represents the actual pain experienced over a given period of time); and whether retrospective pain ratings (memory of pain) were biased by current pain to indicate greater than the average pain experienced by the patient. The horizontal 21-pt box scale emerged as the best scale with respect to psychometrics and validity, regardless of mental status. Little evidence of response perseveration was found on any of the tests. Pain intensity did not vary with mental status. The cognitively impaired group had difficulty with the ratings of least pain, showing a high level of bias in the extent to which memory of pain was influenced by current pain. The investigators concluded that older, cognitively impaired patients are able to rate pain reliably and validly.

Three recent systematic reviews[102-104] and part of a broader guideline for assessing pain in the elderly[23] examined studies of observational methods to assess pain in cognitively impaired adults (Table 4). These instruments rely on examiners to observe facial features and behavior in order to guess how much pain a patient has.

All three reviews concluded that among the numerous scales of nonverbal behavioral pain indicators that currently exist, none are more reliable or valid than others, and none are convincingly appropriate for use in this population. A total of 13 scales were identified in these reviews. Taking all 3 reviews together, the PACSLAC and PAINAD appeared to have the best psychometric properties. Unfortunately, as van Herk and colleagues note, the value of these measures in decision-making is unclear because cutoff values for these scales have not been established.

It is important to note that there is no gold standard for judging the validity of these measures. Most evaluations reported the psychometric properties of these measures rather than their validity.[30] Validity was assessed as agreement with self-report or report of relatives to assess validity; these comparisons are of limited value (if self-report were known to be reliable, there would be little need for using an observational measure.)

Table 4. Pain observation scales. From van Herk et al.[103]

Pain Observation Scale	Target Population	No. of Items	Categories*	Response Category	Score Range
Facial Activity Coding System (FACS)	Cognitively impaired (older) adults	46	1	Frequency and intensity	—
Pain Behavior Method (PBM)	Cognitively impaired (older) adults	5	1, 2, 4	Presence or absence	0–5
Discomfort Scale—Dementia of Alzheimer Type (DS-DAT)	Alzheimer patients	9	1, 2, 4, 6	4-point scale	0–27
DOLOPLUS2	Nonverbal or cognitively impaired older adults	10	1, 2, 3, 4, 5	4-point scale	0–30
Behavior Checklist	Cognitively impaired older adults	20	2, 3, 4, 5, 6	Presence or absence	—
Checklist of Nonverbal Pain Indicators (CNPI)	Cognitively impaired older adults	6	1, 2, 3, 4	Presence or absence	0–6
Assessment for Discomfort in Dementia (ADD)	Patients with moderate to severe dementia	5	1, 2, 3, 4, 5, 6	Presence or absence	—
Pain Assessment in Advanced Dementia (PAINAD)	Patients with (severe) dementia	5	1, 2, 3, 4, 6	3-point scale	0–10
Pain Assessment Tool in Confused Older Adults (PATCOA)	Confused older adults	9	1, 2, 4, 6	Presence or absence	0–9
Pain Assessment for the Dementing Elderly (PADE)	Patients with dementia	24	1, 2, 3, 4, 5, 6	4-point scale and multiple choice	24–96
Pain Assessment Checklist for Seniors with Limited Ability to Communicate (PACSLAC)	Seniors with a limited ability to communicate	60	1, 2, 3, 4, 5, 6	Presence or absence	0–60
Non-Communicative Patient's Pain Assessment Instrument (NOPPAIN)	Noncommunicative patients	17	1, 2, 3, 4, 5	6-point scale	0–30
Abbey Pain Scale	Patients with end-stage dementia	6	1, 2, 3, 4, 5, 6	4-point scale	0–18

Note. *1 = facial expression; 2 = motor behavior; 3 = social behavior or mood; 4 = vocalization; 5 = eat or sleep pattern; 6 = physiological indicators.

Key Question #4. For inpatients with dependencies on tobacco, alcohol, stimulant, marijuana, or opioids, how do differences in assessment and management of acute pain affect clinical outcomes or safety?

Addiction, physical dependence and tolerance are common among inpatients. The ANZCA 2005 report[17] suggested the following for managing acute pain in opioid-tolerant patients:

1) Withdrawal from opioids should be prevented by maintenance of normal preaadmission opioid regimens, or appropriate substitutions with another opioid, or the same opioid via another route. Opioid-tolerant patients are at risk of withdrawal if non-opioid analgesic regimens or tramadol alone are used.
2) Opioid-tolerant patients report higher pain scores and have a lower incidence of opioid-induced nausea and vomiting.
3) Ketamine may reduce opioid requirements in opioid-tolerant patients.
4) Intravenous PCA is a useful modality in opioid-tolerant patients, and larger bolus doses ad a background infusion to replace the usual opioid dose may be needed.
5) Neuraxial opioids can be used although higher doses may be required, and these doses may be inadequate to prevent withdrawal.

6) Patient education regarding prescribed opioids and communication with the primary physician are advisable upon discharge.

The ANZCA 2005 report[17] makes the following suggestions for the management of acute pain in patients with substance abuse disorder:

1) Management of pain in these patients should focus on prevention of withdrawal, effective analgesia, and symptomatic treatment of affective disorders and behavioral alterations.
2) Naltrexone should be stopped at least 24 hours prior to elective surgery, and be replaced by multimodal analgesic regimens.
3) Patients who have completed naltrexone therapy should be regarded as opioid naïve; in the immediate post-treatment phase they may be opioid-sensitivie.
4) Maintenance methadone regimens should be continued where possible
5) Buprenorphine maintenance may be continued; if buprenorphine is ceased prior to surgery, conversion to an alternative opioid is required.
6) There is no cross-tolerance between CNS stimulants and opioids.

The evidence on which these recommendations are based is weak, being derived from case reports, retrospective studies and expert opinion.[17]

How do the assessment and management of acute pain differ between patients on pre-existing opioid therapy and patients with opiate addiction?

In 2001, the American Academy of Pain Medicine, the American Pain Society, and the American Society of Addiction Medicine issued a statement [105] agreeing upon the following definitions:

Tolerance: "Tolerance is a state of adaptation in which exposure to a drug induces changes that result in a diminution of one or more of the drug's effects over time."

Physical Dependence: "Physical dependence is a state of adaptation that often includes tolerance and is manifested by a drug class specific withdrawal syndrome that can be produced by abrupt cessation, rapid dose reduction, decreasing blood level of the drug, and/or administration of an antagonist."

Addiction: "Addiction is a primary, chronic, neurobiological disease, with genetic, psychosocial, and environmental factors influencing its development and manifestations. It is characterized by behaviors that include one or more of the following: impaired control over drug use, compulsive use, continued use despite harm, and craving."

The statement also defined "pseudoaddiction" as "patient behaviors that may occur when pain is undertreated," including a focus on obtaining medications, illicit drug use and deception and other behaviors that may lead clinicians to label them as being "drug seeking." It also said "a patient who is physically dependent on opioids may sometimes continue to use them despite resolution of pain only to avoid withdrawal. Such use does not necessarily reflect addiction."

These definitions are not universally agreed upon, and work to harmonize terminology continues. [106] However, these definitions are consistent with the basic concepts that 1) tolerance and physical dependence are normal responses to opioid therapy, but addiction is not; 2) addictive use of medications is associated with aberrant, destructive behaviors such as "persistent sedation or intoxication due to overuse; increasing functional impairment and other medical complications; psychological manifestations such as irritability, apathy, anxiety, or depression; or adverse legal, economic or social consequences 3) addiction is a multidimensional disease with neurobiological and psychological dimensions. Many guidelines say that a history of addiction to opioids or to alcohol is a relative contraindication for prescribing *chronic* opioids for nonmalignant pain. Guidance on how a history of addiction should influence inpatient management of acute pain is unclear.

The prevalence of addiction among chronic opioid users was unknown.[105] Most studies of the prevalence of addiction among patients with *chronic* pain have used simplistic or outdated criteria for diagnosing addiction, or did not describe their criteria at all.[107] Not surprisingly, estimates of the prevalence of addiction varied wildly, from 0.2% to 50%, depending on the investigators' definition. The apparent prevalence was much lower in studies that used stricter criteria for addiction based on behaviors that are thought to distinguish it from tolerance and physical dependence, and higher in studies that classified patients as addicted if they exhibited "drug-seeking" behavior. While, as a group, the prevalence studies are weak, they do suggest strongly that when a patient on chronic opioid therapy presents with pain, clinicians should not presume that the patient is addicted, and should never diagnose addiction unless there is reason to belief pain control is adequate.

In the literature, there are several lists of signs and symptoms that may be indicators of addiction (as opposed to tolerance and physical dependence.) We found no studies of whether, in acute care settings, clinicians can distinguish addiction from physical dependence or pseudoaddiction. We also found no studies of the discriminant ability of the individual signs and symptoms of addiction, that is, their ability to identify distinct groups of patients for whom different assessment and treatment strategies are most effective.

On the other hand, several instruments intended to screen chronic opioid users for addiction may be helpful in assessing whether relevant signs, symptoms, and behaviors are present. The Pain Medicine Questionnaire and the SOAPP questionnaire have good psychometric properties.[107] The CAGE-AID is a modified CAGE which adapts questions about alcohol to drug use (eg "Have you felt you ought to cut down your drinking *or drug use*?" "Have you felt bad or guilty about your drinking or drug use?" etc.) It has not been tested extensively. None of these instruments has been shown to improve long-term outcomes of chronic nonmalignant pain management, and none has been evaluated in the setting of acute pain in inpatients.

Guidelines for managing post-operative pain specify that initial dosing should be adjusted for patients who take opioids for chronic nonmalignant pain. For the most part, these guidelines for initial dosing have been generalized to patients who have acute pain from other causes, but we did not find any evidence about effectiveness or safety in the target population for this report.

CONCLUSIONS

The results of the systematic evidence review, including the type and quality of evidence for each key question, are summarized in Table 5 below.

Table 5. Summary of Systematic Evidence Review, Key Question 1. How do differences in timing and frequency of assessment, severity of pain, and follow-up of pain affect choice of treatment, clinical outcomes, and safety?

KQ#	Key question	Type of Evidence	Grade of Evidence	Comments
1a	In medical inpatients with acute pain, does routine assessment of pain affect choice of treatment, clinical outcomes, and safety?	None	**GRADE Very Low** = Any estimate of effect is very uncertain.	We found no evidence that directly linked the timing, frequency, or choice of measure for assessment with the timeliness, choice, or safety of treatment specifically in medical inpatients. Older studies demonstrated that observational assessment of pain by a nurse or physician is inaccurate.
1b	Does the choice of assessment measure affect choice of treatment, clinical outcomes, and safety?	1 descriptive study in cancer patients	**GRADE Low** = Further research is very likely to have an important impact on our confidence in the estimate of effect and is likely to change the estimate.	Within a program of routine assessment of pain, we found no studies of how the choice of assessment measure affects the choice of treatment, clinical outcomes, or safety. Most studies focus on the psychometric qualities and ease of administration of each method. In cancer patients, there is fair evidence from one observational study that opioid-related oversedation and other adverse effects increased substantially after implementation of pain assessment on a numerical scale routinely with other vital signs.
1c	Do protocols for assessing pain improve outcomes?	None	**Very Low**	In most cases, these protocols are part of larger, institution-wide strategies to improve pain management. We found no evaluations that could isolate the effect of algorithms, preprinted orders, clinical pathways, or other protocols for assessing pain in the target population.
1d	Are there gaps in quality even when pain is assessed routinely?	5 descriptive studies in the ED	**GRADE Moderate** = Further research is likely to have an important impact on our confidence in the estimate of effect and may change the estimate.	*3 chart review studies in the ED setting found that gaps in quality that remain after institution of system changes. Having a lower-priority triage score, older age, and diagnostic uncertainty were factors associated with delay or lower likelihood of receiving analgesia. In a study of patients with acute abdomen in an ED with direct access to on-call surgical service, females, less severe pain, and daytime admissions predicted delays in analgesia, despite the elimination of referral delay.*
1e	*Specific condition: nonsurgical abdominal pain*	*1 systematic review and meta-analysis of randomized trials and 1 additional trial*	*GRADE High = Further research is very unlikely to change our confidence on the estimate of effect.*	*Opioid administration has a negligible impact on clinical management of acute abdominal pain.*

Summary of Key Question 2. How do the timing and route of administration of pain interventions compare in effectiveness, adverse effects, and safety in inpatient care settings?

KQ#	Key question	Type of Evidence	Grade of Evidence	Comments
2a	Do acute pain management teams and other institutional initiatives improve effectiveness, adverse effects, and safety in medical inpatients?	1 uncontrolled systemwide intervention and 1 controlled trial	Moderate	1 uncontrolled collaborative VHA/IHI study of institution-wide strategies showed measurable improvements in the prevalence of severe pain, frequency of assessment and documentation of plan of care, and provision of patient education on pain management. A controlled trial of a multifaceted intervention achieved increased assessment of pain but did not alter pain intensity or duration.
2b	Do acute pain management teams and other institutional initiatives improve effectiveness, adverse effects, and safety in other settings?	2 systematic reviews of before-after or uncontrolled studies	Low	Most primary studies in these reviews were in postoperative or cancer pain, and were uncontrolled. While pain management teams and other system-wide interventions improved the timeliness and frequency of pain assessment, the findings were mixed for improvement in pain outcomes. In controlled studies, Acute Pain Services reduced pain intensity and improved functional ability, although the magnitude of these effects was not always clinically important.
2c	How does coordination with the patient's primary care physician affect outcomes?	None	Very Low	*We found no evidence about the value of coordinating care with the patient's primary care physician.*
2d	How does the choice of treatment modality affect effectiveness, adverse effects, and safety in inpatient care settings?	None	Very Low	*We found no evidence on the comparative effectiveness of different agents and methods of administration in general inpatients.*
2e	Effectiveness and safety of patient-controlled analgesia (PCA)	3 controlled trials and 1 cohort study	Low	*There is almost no information on the use or safety of PCA in a medical ward setting. Most of the evidence on the adverse effects of PCA was derived from the experience of patients with postoperative or chronic conditions.*

		Moderate	(1) NSAIDs provide effective analgesia for acute renal colic, and act more quickly through the IV route than by IM or PR 2) Opioids provide analgesia that is equivalent to NSAIDs but result in a higher incidence of vomiting and other adverse events, particularly pethidine 3) Hydromorphone provided superior pain relief and led to fewer hospital admissions compared with meperidine in one study. Many studies excluded patients who had negative followup investigations for biliary stone or renal calculi, which may limit the applicability of findings to all patients presenting with pain from these suspected causes.
	Specific conditions: renal colic and biliary stone pain	Renal colic studies: 3 RCTs comparing route of NSAID administration; 1 systematic review of NSAIDS vs. opioids; 1 RCT of hydromorphone; 1 study of hydromorphone in biliary pain	
2g	Specific conditions: phantom limb pain	1 systematic review of controlled trials	*Low*	*Overall there is a paucity of evidence to guide specific specific treatment of phantom limb pain. The evidence on preemptive epidurals, early regional nerve blocks, and mechanical vibratory stimulation provides inconsistent support for these treatments. Single studies showed evidence of the effectiveness of various therapies (calcitonin, morphine, ketamine, gabapentin, and sensory discrimination training), and perioperative studies of ketamine and epidural analgesia showed reduced incidence of phantom limb pain, but these studies were limited by small sample size.*

Summary of Key Questions 3 and 4.

KQ#	Key question	Type of Evidence	Grade of Evidence	Comments
3	For inpatients with impaired self-report due to any of several factors, including delirium or confusion, pre-existing severe dementia, closed head injury, stroke, and psychosis, how do differences in assessment and management of acute pain affect clinical outcomes or safety?	3 systematic reviews of descriptive and cross-sectional evaluations of assessment instruments; no study designs were excluded	Low	Most studies were conducted in nursing homes in patients with dementia, and focused on assessment. Delirium is a more common cause of cognitive impairment in the medical inpatient setting, and we identified no studies of pain assessment or management in patients with delirium. All 3 reviews concluded that among the numerous scales of nonverbal behavioral pain indicators in use, none are more reliable or valid than others, and none are convincingly appropriate for use in this population. The reviews included a total of 13 scales, and the PACSLAC and PAINAD appear to have the best psychometric properties. The value of these measures in decision-making is unclear, however, because cutoff values for these scales have not been established. We found no studies that directly linked differences in assessment and management with clinical outcomes or safety in this subgroup of patients.
4a	For inpatients with dependencies on tobacco, alcohol, stimulant, marijuana, or opioids, how do differences in assessment and management of acute pain affect clinical outcomes or safety?	Case reports, retrospective studies, and expert opinions identified by a systematic search	Low	*Guidelines for managing acute pain in opioid-tolerant patients and patients with substance abuse disorder are based on case reports, retrospective studies, and expert opinion were compiled in a good-quality systematic review. The evidence on which these recommendations are based is weak, however, being derived from case reports, retrospective studies and expert opinion*
4b	*How do the assessment and mangement of acute pain differ between patients on pre-existing opioid therapy and patients with opiate addiction?*	*None*	*Very Low*	*Definitions for tolerance, physical dependence, and addiction, and pseudoaddiction are not universally agreed upon, and estimates of the prevalence of addiction in patients with chronic pain varied widely, from 0.2% to 50%. We found no studies of whether in acute care settings, clinicians can distinguish addiction from physical dependence or pseudoaddiction. We also found no studies of the discriminant ability of individual signs and symptoms of addiction to identify distinct groups of patients for whom different assessment and treatment strategies are most effective. Guidelines for managing post-operative pain specify that initial dosing should be adjusted for patients who take opioids for chronic nonmalignant pain, and while these guidelines for initial dosing have been generalized to patients who have acute pain from other causes, we did not find any evidence about effectiveness or safety in the target population.*

Recommendations for future research

Pain is a prevalent problem for medical inpatients, and research has not addressed this setting effectively. The lack of evidence suggests that the VA should characterize current practice, avoid overly prescriptive standards, and emphasize a robust research agenda. Given that pain intensity is used widely, and that outpatient research raises some questions about the accuracy and relevance of single item screening for pain to improved patient outcomes, veterans might benefit from clinical research that:

1) Tests use of pain intensity along with other approaches (automated nurse / physician alerts, expanded screening items / paradigms, patient direct-triggered nurse / physician alerts) to better link screening to intervention. Psychometric evaluation is needed as one aspect of this research.
2) Draws upon quality improvement research to evaluate the efficacy of key intervention components.
3) Evaluates different initial treatment intensities including the clinical effectiveness and safety of PCA, but not excluding high intensity oral regimes (which are used in lieu of PCA in places such as Australia). These studies should stress the evaluation of alternative follow-up strategies and ascertain the risk / benefit and ceiling effects of alternative approaches to medical pain management.
4) Specifically addresses basic clinical science of pain in delirium, severe mental illness (such as schizophrenia which you highlight) and dementia (such as identifying a 'gold standard' for validity – e.g., fMRI vs. observation), and clinical studies that address 1-3 should not exclude veterans with substance abuse disorder. Furthermore, studies that examine treatment in those populations and that include outcomes relevant to prior abuse such as triggering of recurrent abuse, dysphoria, etc., are needed.
5) Evaluates performance measures that go beyond assessment to include prompt treatment and successful alleviation of pain in the medical inpatient setting (see Table 6).

Additional recommendations pertinent to VA care can be found in Buffum et al.[97]

Table 6. Examples of indicators for measuring aspects of pain management

Performance measure	Developed for population/setting	Numerator	Denominator
Assessment and diagnosis			
Percentage of patients with documented assessment for pain using standardized tool on admission[108]	Long-term care setting	Number with documented admission assessment for pain using standardized tool	All patients
Percentage of patients with documented care plan for acute or chronic pain[108]	Long-term care setting	Number with documented care plan for acute or chronic pain	All patients with reported pain
Percentage of patients receiving physical exam to assess for causes of pain[108]	Long-term care setting	Number receiving physical exam to assess for causes of pain	All patients with reported pain
Percentage with cognitive and language problems receiving targeted pain assessment[108]	Long-term care setting	Number with cognitive and language problems receiving targeted pain assessment	Patients with diagnosed cognitive and/or language deficit
Percentage with periodic documented assessment by nursing staff of effectiveness of pain management[108]	Long-term care setting	Number with periodic documented assessment by nursing staff of effectiveness of pain management	Patients with reported pain
Percentage with periodic documented assessment of effectiveness of pain management by medical doctor (MD)[108]	Long-term care setting	Number with periodic documented assessment of effectiveness of pain management by medical doctor (MD)	Patients with reported pain
Percentage with documented complete assessment of pain covering all pertinent components of pain[108]	Long-term care setting	Number with documented complete assessment of pain covering all pertinent components of pain	All patients with reported pain
Screening for pain[109]	Vulnerable elders (aged 65+)	Number of patients screened for chronic pain in initial evaluation	All vulnerable elders
Screening for depression[109]	Vulnerable elders (aged 65+)	Number of patients screened for depression	Vulnerable elders with presenting with chronic pain
Treatment/ management			
Percentage with documented absence of pain symptoms after treatment[108]	Long-term care setting	Number with documented absence of pain symptoms after treatment	All patients with reported pain who received treatment
Percentage with documented reduction of pain symptoms[108]	Long-term care setting	Number of patients with documented reduction of pain symptoms	All patients with reported pains
Percentage of patients	Long-term care	Number of patients with	All patients receiving

with orders for not recommended drugs[108]	setting	orders for not recommended drugs	medications to treat pain
Percentage of patients with appropriate treatment for pain[108]	Long-term care setting	Number of patients with appropriate treatment for pain	All patients with reported pain
Percentage of patients prescribed narcotics for pain with appropriate bowel management program in place[108]	Long-term care setting	Number of patients prescribed narcotics with appropriate bowel management in place	All patients receiving narcotics to treat pain
Percentage with adverse drug reactions (ADRs) to pain medications[108]	Long-term care setting	Number of patients with adverse drug reactions (ADRs) related to pain medications	All patients receiving pain medication
Percentage with controlled adverse drug reactions (ADRs) to pain medications[108]	Long-term care setting	Number with controlled adverse drug reactions (ADRs) to pain medications	All patients with reported pain receiving pain medication who had an adverse drug reaction (ADR)
Addressing risks of NSAIDs[109]	Vulnerable elders (aged 65+)	Number of patients whose medical record indicates whether s/he has a history of peptic ulcer disease, and if a history is present, documentation of justification of NSAID use	All vulnerable elders who have been prescribed a cyclooxygenase nonselective NSAID for the treatment of chronic pain
Constipation with opioid use[109]	Vulnerable elders (aged 65+)	Number of vulnerable elders offered a bowel regimen, or whose medical record documents the potential for constipation or explains why bowel treatment is not needed.	All vulnerable elders treated with opioids for chronic pain
Meperidine not used[109]	Vulnerable elders (aged 65+)	Number of patients requiring analgesia who were not given meperidine	All vulnerable elders who require analgesia
Percentage who reported how often their pain was controlled[110]	Adult inpatients	The number of respondents from the denominator who indicated "Always," "Usually", "Sometimes," or "Never" on the two questions regarding their experiences with control of their pain	Hospital inpatients with an admission during the reporting period who answered the "Pain Management" questions on the CAHPS Hospital Survey

REFERENCES

1. Ngo AL, Guiang R. Acute pain management. In: Boswell MV, Cole BE, eds. *Weiner's pain management: A practical guide for clinicians, 7th edition*. Boca Raton: CRC Press; 2006.
2. Dix P, Sandhar B, Murdoch J, MacIntyre PA. Pain on medical wards in a district general hospital. *British Journal of Anaesthesia*. 2004;92(2):235-237.
3. Johnson L, Regaard A, Herrington N. Pain in general medical patients: an audit. In: Dostrovsky JO CD, Koltzenburg, eds. , ed. *Proceedings of the 10th World Congress of Pain. Progress in Pain Research and Management. .* Vol 24. Seattle: : IASP Press; 2003.
4. Melotti RM, Samolsky-Dekel BG, Ricchi E, et al. Pain prevalence and predictors among inpatients in a major Italian teaching hospital. A baseline survey towards a pain free hospital. *European Journal of Pain: Ejp*. Oct 2005;9(5):485-495.
5. Vallano A, Malouf J, Payrulet P, Banos JE. Prevalence of pain in adults admitted to Catalonian hospitals: a cross-sectional study. *Eur J Pain*. Nov 2006;10(8):721-731.
6. Visentin M, Zanolin E, Trentin L, Sartori S, de Marco R. Prevalence and treatment of pain in adults admitted to Italian hospitals. *European Journal of Pain: Ejp*. Feb 2005;9(1):61-67.
7. *The Integrated Approach to the Management of Pain. NIH Consensus Statement*: National Institutes of Health; 1986.
8. Warfield CA, Kahn CH. Acute pain management. Programs in U.S. hospitals and experiences and attitudes among U.S. adults. *Anesthesiology*. Nov 1995;83(5):1090-1094.
9. Morrison RS, Magaziner J, McLaughlin MA, et al. The impact of post-operative pain on outcomes following hip fracture. *Pain*. Jun 2003;103(3):303-311.
10. Anonymous. *Acute Pain Management: Operative or Medical Procedures and Trauma*: Agency for Health Care Policy and Research; February 1992 1992. AHCPR Publication No. 92-0032.
11. *Management of cancer pain*: Agency for Health Care Policy and Research; February 1992 1994. AHCPR Publication No. 92-0032.
12. Shojania KG, Duncan BW, McDonald KM. *Making Health Care Safer: A Critical Analysis of Patient Safety Practices.*: Agency for Healthcare Research and Quality; 2001. AHRQ Publication No. 01-E058.
13. Cleeland CS, Reyes-Gibby CC, Schall M, et al. Rapid improvement in pain management: the Veterans Health Administration and the institute for healthcare improvement collaborative. *Clin J Pain*. Sep-Oct 2003;19(5):298-305.
14. Craine M, Kerns RD. Pain Management Improvement Strategies in the Veteran's Health Administration. *APS Bulletin*. 2003;13(5).
15. McMillan SC, Tittle M, Hagan S, Laughlin J. Management of Pain and Pain-Related Symptoms in Hospitalized Veterans With Cancer. *Cancer Nursing*. 2000;23(5):327-336.
16. Kerns RD, Booss J, Bryan M, et al. Veterans Health Administration National Pain Management Strategy: Update and Future Directions. *APS Bulletin*. 2006;16(1).

17. Australian and New Zealand College of Anaesthetists and Faculty of Pain Medicine. Acute Pain Management: Scientific Evidence, 2nd edition. *Melbourne: Australian and New Zealand College of Anaesthetists.* 2005.

18. Macintyre PE, Schug SA, Scott DA. Acute pain management: the evidence grows. An Australian document now has an important role in acute pain management worldwide. *Medical Journal of Australia* 2006;184(3):101-2.

19. Merlin T, Hodgkinson B, Macintyre PE, Ludbrook G, Hiller JE. Institutional approaches to pain assessment and management (008PAI). A systematic literature review. *Health Technology Assessment Database.* 2003(1).

20. *ICSI Health Care Guideline: Assessment and Management of Acute Pain, 5th Edition* 2006.

21. *Pain: Current Understanding of Assessment, Management, and Treatments* Joint Commission on Accreditation of Healthcare Organizations; 2001.

22. *Improving the quality of pain management through measurement and action*: Joint Commission on Accreditation of Healthcare Organizations; 2003.

23. Hadjistavropoulos T, Herr K, Turk DC, et al. An Interdisciplinary Expert Consensus Statement on Assessment of Pain in Older Persons. *Clinical Journal of Pain.* 2007;23 Supplement 1:S1-S43.

24. Harris RP, Helfand M, Woolf SH, et al. Current methods of the US Preventive Services Task Force: a review of the process. *American Journal of Preventive Medicine.* Apr 2001;20(3 Suppl):21-35.

25. Mora B. Giorni E. Dobrovits M. Barker R. Lang T. Gore C. Kober A. Transcutaneous electrical nerve stimulation: an effective treatment for pain caused by renal colic in emergency care. *Journal of Urology. 175(5):1737-41; discussion 1741, 2006 May.*

26. Frasco PE, Sprung J, Trentman TL. The Impact of the Joint Commission for Accreditation of Healthcare Organizations Pain Initiative on Perioperative Opiate Consumption and Recovery Room Length of Stay. *Anesth Analg.* January 1, 2005 2005;100(1):162-168.

27. Nelson BP, Cohen D, Lander O, Crawford N, Viccellio AW, Singer AJ. Mandated pain scales improve frequency of ED analgesic administration. *American Journal of Emergency Medicine.* Nov 2004;22(7):582-585.

28. Luger TJ, Lederer W, Gassner M, Lockinger A, Ulmer H, Lorenz IH. Acute pain is underassessed in out-of-hospital emergencies. *Academic Emergency Medicine.* Jun 2003;10(6):627-632.

29. Carey SJ, Turpin C, Smith J, Whatley J, Haddox D. Improving pain management in an acute care setting. The Crawford Long Hospital of Emory University experience. *Orthopaedic Nursing.* Jul-Aug 1997;16(4):29-36.

30. Peters ML, Patijn J, Lame I. Pain Assessment in Younger and Older Pain Patients: Psychometric Properties and Patient Preference of Five Commonly Used Measures of Pain Intensity. *Pain Medicine.* 2007;8(7):601-610.

31. Morrison RS, Ahronheim JC, Morrison GR, et al. Pain and discomfort associated with common hospital procedures and experiences. *Journal of Pain and Symptom Management.* 1998;15(2):91-101.

32. Jaeschke R, Singer J, Guyatt GH. Measurement of health status. Ascertaining the minimal clinically important difference. *Control Clin Trials.* 1989;10(4):407-415.

33.   Grant MD, Samson D. Special Report: Measuring and Reporting Pain Outcomes in Randomized Controlled Trials. *TEC Assessment Program.* 2006;21(11).

34.   Vila H, Jr., Smith RA, Augustyniak MJ, et al. The Efficacy and Safety of Pain Management Before and After Implementation of Hospital-Wide Pain Management Standards: Is Patient Safety Compromised by Treatment Based Solely on Numerical Pain Ratings? *Anesth. Analg.* August 1, 2005 2005;101(2):474-480.

35.   Mularski RA, White-Chu F, Overbay D, Miller L, Asch SM, Ganzini L. Measuring Pain as the 5th Vital Sign Does Not Improve Quality of Pain Management. *Journal of General Internal Medicine.* 2006;21(6):607-612.

36.   Krebs EE, Carey TS, Weinberger M. Accuracy of the Pain Numeric Rating Scale as a Screening Test in Primary Care. *J Gen Intern Med.* 2007;21(10):1453-1458.

37.   Tanabe P, Buschmann M. A prospective study of ED pain management practices and the patient's perspective. *Journal of Emergency Nursing.* Jun 1999;25(3):171-177.

38.   Blank FS, Mader TJ, Wolfe J, Keyes M, Kirschner R, Provost D. Adequacy of pain assessment and pain relief and correlation of patient satisfaction in 68 ED fast-track patients. *Journal of Emergency Nursing.* Aug 2001;27(4):327-334.

39.   Grant PS. Analgesia delivery in the ED. *American Journal of Emergency Medicine.* Nov 2006;24(7):806-809.

40.   Jones JB. Assessment of pain management skills in emergency medicine residents: the role of a pain education program. *Journal of Emergency Medicine.* Mar-Apr 1999;17(2):349-354.

41.   Kelly AM. A process approach to improving pain management in the emergency department: development and evaluation. *Journal of Accident & Emergency Medicine.* May 2000;17(3):185-187.

42.   Fosnocht DE, Swanson ER. Use of a triage pain protocol in the ED. *American Journal of Emergency Medicine.* Sep 2007;25(7):791-793.

43.   Arendts G, Fry M. Factors associated with delay to opiate analgesia in emergency departments. *Journal of Pain.* Sep 2006;7(9):682-686.

44.   Hwang U, Richardson LD, Sonuyi TO, Morrison RS. The effect of emergency department crowding on the management of pain in older adults with hip fracture. *Journal of the American Geriatrics Society.* Feb 2006;54(2):270-275.

45.   Pines JM, Hollander JE. Emergency department crowding is associated with poor care for patients with severe pain. *Annals of Emergency Medicine.* Jan 2008;51(1):1-5; discussion 6-7.

46.   Graber MA, Ely JW, Clarke S, Kurtz S, Weir R. Informed consent and general surgeons' attitudes toward the use of pain medication in the acute abdomen. *American Journal of Emergency Medicine.* Mar 1999;17(2):113-116.

47.   Attard AR, Corlett MJ, Kidner NJ, Leslie AP, Fraser IA. Safety of early pain relief for acute abdominal pain. *BMJ.* 1992;305:554-556.

48.   Pace S, Burke T. Intravenous morphine for early pain relief in patients with acute abdominal pain. *Academic emergency medicine : official journal of the Society for Academic Emergency Medicine.* 1996;3(12):1086-1092.

49.   McHale PM, LoVecchio F. Narcotic analgesia in the acute abdomen--a review of prospective trials. *Eur J Emerg Med.* Jun 2001;8(2):131-136.

50.   Nissman SA, Kaplan LJ, Mann BD. Critically reappraising the literature-driven practice of analgesia administration for acute abdominal pain in the emergency room prior to surgical evaluation. *American Journal of Surgery.* Apr 2003;185(4):291-296.

51.   Ranji SR, Goldman LE, Simel DL, Shojania KG. Do opiates affect the clinical evaluation of patients with acute abdominal pain? *JAMA.* Oct 11 2006;296(14):1764-1774.

52.   Bijur PE, Berard A, Esses D, Nestor J, Schechter C, Gallagher EJ. Lack of influence of patient self-report of pain intensity on administration of opioids for suspected long-bone fractures. *Journal of Pain.* Jun 2006;7(6):438-444.

53.   Shabbir J, Ridgway PF, Lynch K, et al. Administration of analgesia for acute abdominal pain sufferers in the accident and emergency setting. *European Journal of Emergency Medicine.* Dec 2004;11(6):309-312.

54.   Morrison RS, Meier DE, Fischberg D, et al. Improving the management of pain in hospitalized adults. *Archives of Internal Medicine.* May 8 2006;166(9):1033-1039.

55.   Goldberg GR, Morrison RS. Pain management in hospitalized cancer patients: a systematic review`. *J Clin Oncology.* 2007;25(13):1792-1801.

56.   White PF. Use of patient-controlled analgesia for management of acute pain. *JAMA.* Jan 8 1988;259(2):243-247.

57.   Fulda GJ, Giberson F, Fagraeus L. A prospective randomized trial of nebulized morphine compared with patient-controlled analgesia morphine in the management of acute thoracic pain. *Journal of Trauma-Injury Infection & Critical Care.* Aug 2005;59(2):383-388; discussion 389-390.

58.   Evans E, Turley N, Robinson N, Clancy M. Randomised controlled trial of patient controlled analgesia compared with nurse delivered analgesia in an emergency department. *Emergency Medicine Journal.* Jan 2005;22(1):25-29.

59.   Moon MR, Luchette FA, Gibson SW, et al. Prospective, randomized comparison of epidural versus parenteral opioid analgesia in thoracic trauma. *Annals of Surgery.* May 1999;229(5):684-691; discussion 691-682.

60.   Wu CL, Jani ND, Perkins FM, Barquist E. Thoracic epidural analgesia versus intravenous patient-controlled analgesia for the treatment of rib fracture pain after motor vehicle crash. *Journal of Trauma-Injury Infection & Critical Care.* Sep 1999;47(3):564-567.

61.   Liu SS, Wu CL. The Effect of Analgesic Technique on Postoperative Patient-Reported Outcomes Including Analgesia: A Systematic Review. *Anesth Analg.* September 1, 2007 2007;105(3):789-808.

62.   Liu SS, Wu CL. Effect of Postoperative Analgesia on Major Postoperative Complications: A Systematic Update of the Evidence. *Anesth Analg.* March 1, 2007 2007;104(3):689-702.

63.   Bainbridge D, Martin JE, Cheng DC. Patient-controlled versus nurse-controlled analgesia after cardiac surgery--a meta-analysis. *Canadian Journal of Anaesthesia.* May 2006;53(5):492-499.

64.   Block BM, Liu SS, Rowlingson AJ, Cowan AR, Cowan JA, Jr., Wu CL. Efficacy of Postoperative Epidural Analgesia: A Meta-analysis. *JAMA.* November 12, 2003 2003;290(18):2455-2463.

65. Walder B, Schafer M, Henzi I, Tramer MR. Efficacy and safety of patient-controlled opioid analgesia for acute postoperative pain. A quantitative systematic review. *Acta Anaesthesiologica Scandinavica.* Aug 2001;45(7):795-804.

66. Hudcova J, McNicol E, Quah C, Lau J, Carr DB. Patient controlled opioid analgesia versus conventional opioid analgesia for postoperative pain. *Cochrane Database of Systematic Reviews.* 2007(2).

67. Hudcova J, McNicol E, Quah C, Lau J, Carr DB. Patient controlled opioid analgesia versus conventional opioid analgesia for postoperative pain. *Cochrane Database of Systematic Reviews.* 2006(4):CD003348.

68. Tziavrangos E, Schug SA. Regional anaesthesia and perioperative outcome. *Current Opinion in Anaesthesiology.* Oct 2006;19(5):521-525.

69. Werawatganon T, Charuluxanun S. Patient controlled intravenous opioid analgesia versus continuous epidural analgesia for pain after intra-abdominal surgery. *Cochrane Database of Systematic Reviews.* 2007(2).

70. Werawatganon T, Charuluxanun S. Patient controlled intravenous opioid analgesia versus continuous epidural analgesia for pain after intra-abdominal surgery. *Cochrane Database of Systematic Reviews.* 2005(1):CD004088.

71. Macintyre PE. Safety and efficacy of patient-controlled analgesia. *British Journal of Anaesthesia.* Jul 2001;87(1):36-46.

72. Hagle ME, Lehr VT, Brubakken K, Shippee A. Respiratory depression in adult patients with intravenous patient-controlled analgesia. *Orthopaedic Nursing.* Jan-Feb 2004;23(1):18-27; quiz 28-19.

73. Ashburn MA, Love G, Pace NL. Respiratory-related critical events with intravenous patient-controlled analgesia. *Clinical Journal of Pain.* Mar 1994;10(1):52-56.

74. Tramer MR, Williams JE, Carroll D, Wiffen PJ, Moore RA, McQuay HJ. Comparing analgesic efficacy of non-steroidal anti-inflammatory drugs given by different routes in acute and chronic pain: a qualitative systematic review. *Acta Anaesthesiologica Scandinavica.* Jan 1998;42(1):71-79.

75. Nelson CE, Nylander C, Olsson AM, Olsson R, Pettersson BA, Wallstrom I. Rectal v. intravenous administration of indomethacin in the treatment of renal colic. *Acta Chirurgica Scandinavica.* Apr 1988;154(4):253-255.

76. Nissen I, Birke H, Olsen JB, et al. Treatment of ureteric colic. Intravenous versus rectal administration of indomethacin. *British Journal of Urology.* Jun 1990;65(6):576-579.

77. Muriel-Villoria C, Zungri-Telo E, Diaz-Curiel M, et al. Comparison of the onset and duration of the analgesic effect of dipyrone, 1 or 2 g, by the intramuscular or intravenous route, in acute renal colic. *European Journal of Clinical Pharmacology.* 1995;48(2):103-107.

78. Holdgate A, Pollock T. Nonsteroidal anti-inflammatory drugs (NSAIDS) versus opioids for acute renal colic. *Cochrane Database of Systematic Reviews.* 2007(2).

79. Quigley C. Hydromorphone for acute and chronic pain. *Cochrane Database of Systematic Reviews.* 2007(2).

80. Jasani NB, O'Conner RE, Bouzoukis JK. Comparison of hydromorphone and meperidine for ureteral colic. *Academic Emergency Medicine.* Nov-Dec 1994;1(6):539-543.

81. Uden P, Starck CJ, Berger T. Comparison of indomethacin and dihydromorphinone in acute, biliary stone pain. *Current Ther Res.* 1984;36(6):1228-1234.

82. Halbert J, Crotty M. Evidence for the optimal management of acute and chronic phantom pain: a systematic review. *Clin J Pain* 2002;18(2):84-92.

83. Sherman RA, Sherman CJ, Gall NG. A survey of current phantom limb pain treatment in the United States. *Pain.* 1980;8:85-99.

84. Jaeger H, Maier C. Calcitonin in phantom limb pain: a double-blind study. *Pain.* Jan 1992;48(1):21-27.

85. Nikolajsen L, Hansen CL, Nielsen J, Keller J, Arendt-Nielsen L, Jensen TS. The effect of ketamine on phantom pain: a central neuropathic disorder maintained by peripheral input. *Pain.* Sep 1996;67(1):69-77.

86. Huse E, Larbig W, Flor H, Birbaumer N. The effect of opioids on phantom limb pain and cortical reorganization. *Pain.* Feb 1 2001;90(1-2):47-55.

87. Wu CL, Tella P, Staats PS, et al. Analgesic effects of intravenous lidocaine and morphine on postamputation pain: a randomized double-blind, active placebo-controlled, crossover trial. *Anesthesiology.* Apr 2002;96(4):841-848.

88. Bone M, Critchley P, Buggy DJ. Gabapentin in postamputation phantom limb pain: a randomized, double-blind, placebo-controlled, cross-over study. *Regional Anesthesia & Pain Medicine.* Sep-Oct 2002;27(5):481-486.

89. Dertwinkel R, Henrichs C, Senne I, et al. Prevention of severe phantom limb pain by perioperative administration of ketamine - an observational study. *Acute Pain.* 2002;4:9-13.

90. Hayes C, Armstrong-Brown A, Burstal R. Perioperative intravenous ketamine infusion for the prevention of persistent post-amputation pain: a randomized, controlled trial. *Anaesthesia & Intensive Care.* Jun 2004;32(3):330-338.

91. Gehling M, Tryba M. [Prophylaxis of phantom pain: is regional analgesia ineffective?]. *Schmerz.* Jan 2003;17(1):11-19.

92. Flor H, Denke C, Schaefer M, Grusser S. Effect of sensory discrimination training on cortical reorganisation and phantom limb pain. *Lancet.* Jun 2 2001;357(9270):1763-1764.

93. Cook AK, Niven CA, Downs MG. Assessing the pain of people with cognitive impairment. *International Journal of Geriatric Psychiatry.* Jun 1999;14(6):421-425.

94. Weiner D, Peterson B, Ladd K, McConnell E, Keefe F. Pain in nursing home residents: An exploration of prevalence, staff perspectives, and practical aspects of measurement. *Clin J Pain.* 1999;15(2):92-101.

95. Parmelee P. Pain complaints and cognitive status among elderly institution residents. . *Journal of the American Geriatrics Society.* 1993;41(5):517-522.

96. Pautex S, Michon A, Guedira M, et al. Pain in severe dementia: self-assessment or observational scales?. *Journal of the American Geriatrics Society.* 2006;54(7):1040-1045.

97. Buffum MD, Hutt E, Chang VT, Craine MH, Snow AL. Cognitive impairment and pain management: Review of issues and challenges. *Journal of Rehabilitation Research & Development.* 2007;44(2):315-330.

98. Assessing Pain in the Patient with Impaired Communication: A Consensus Statement from the VHA National Pain Management Strategy Coordinating Committee. In: Affairs V, ed; 2004.

99. Pautex S, Herrmann F, Le Lous P, Fabjan M, Michel JP, Gold G. Feasibility and reliability of four pain self-assessment scales and correlation with an observational rating scale in hospitalized elderly demented patients. *. Journals of Gerontology Series A-Biological Sciences & Medical Sciences.* Apr 2005;60(4):524-529.

100. Defrin R, Lotan M, Pick CG. The evaluation of acute pain in individuals with cognitive impairment: a differential effect of the level of impairment. *Pain.* Oct 2006;124(3):312-320.

101. Chibnall JT, Tait RC. Pain assessment in cognitively impaired and unimpaired older adults: a comparison of four scales. *Pain.* May 2001;92(1-2):173-186.

102. Herr K, Bjoro K, Decker S. Tools for assessment of pain in nonverbal older adults with dementia: a state-of-the-science review. *Journal of Pain & Symptom Management.* Feb 2006;31(2):170-192.

103. van Herk R, van Dijk M, Baar FP, Tibboel D, de Wit R. Observation scales for pain assessment in older adults with cognitive impairments or communication difficulties. *Nurs Res.* 2007;56(1):34-43.

104. Zwakhalen SMG, Hamers JPH, Abu-Saad HH, Berger MPF. Pain in elderly people with severe dementia: a systematic review of behavioural pain assessment tools. *BMC Geriatrics.* 2006;6:3.

105. Definitions Related to the Use of Opioids for the Treatment of Pain. http://www.ampainsoc.org/advocacy/opioids2.htm. Accessed December 10, 2007, 2007.

106. Savage SR, Joranson DE, Covington EC, Schnoll SH, Heit HA, Gilson AM. Definitions related to the medical use of opioids: evolution towards universal agreement. *. J Pain Symptom Manage.* 2003;26:655–667.

107. Hojsted J, Sjogren P. Addiction to opioids in chronic pain patients: A literature review. *European Journal of Pain.* 2007;11(5):490-518.

108. American Medical Directors Association. We care: tool kit for implementation of the clinical practice guideline for pain management. Columbia (MD): American Medical Directors Association (AMDA); 2004.

109. ACOVE quality indicators. Assessing the Care of Vulnerable Elders Project. Rand Health, Santa Monica, California. Chodosh J, Ferrell BA, Shekelle PG, et al. Quality indicators for pain management in vulnerable elders. Ann Intern Med. 2001: 135 (8pt2):641-758, 731-738.

110. Agency for Healthcare Research and Quality (AHRQ). CAHPS hospital survey. Rockville (MD): Agency for Healthcare Research and Quality (AHRQ); 2006 Feb 1. 4 p. Centers for Medicare & Medicaid Services (CMS). HCAHPS survey [http://www.hcahpsonline.org]. Baltimore (MD): Centers for Medicare & Medicaid Services (CMS)

APPENDIX A. Search Strategy

Database: Ovid MEDLINE(R) <1996 to April Week 1 2007>
Search Strategy:

----

1   Analgesia/ or Analgesics, Opioid/ or Pain/ or Anti-Inflammatory Agents, Non-Steroidal/ or acute pain.mp. or Pain Measurement/ or Analgesics/ (89900)
2   Meta-Analysis/ or "Review Literature"/ or systematic review.mp. (15321)
3   1 and 2 (661)
4   limit 3 to english language (596)
5   from 4 keep 1-596 (596)

Targeted search strategy for primary studies on KQ1:
Database: Ovid MEDLINE(R) <1950 to July Week 2 2007>
Search Strategy:

----

1   exp Pain/ (212174)
2   exp Pain Measurement/ (31393)
3   ((assess$ or measur$) adj3 pain$).mp. [mp=title, original title, abstract, name of substance word, subject heading word] (37632)
4   acute pain$.mp. (2813)
5   1 or 2 or 3 or 4 (226036)
6   exp Hospitalization/ (104116)
7   exp Inpatients/ (6381)
8   exp patient admission/ (12978)
9   exp Emergency Medical Services/ (60608)
10   6 or 7 or 8 or 9 (163418)
11   5 and 10 (5687)
12   exp Time/ (845509)
13   11 and 12 (778)
14   limit 13 to (humans and english language) (657)
15   from 14 keep 1-657 (657)

Targeted search strategy for primary studies on the use of PCA in non-surgical settings, for KQ2:
Database: Ovid MEDLINE(R) <1950 to July Week 3 2007>
Search Strategy:

----

1   Analgesia, Patient-Controlled/ (2508)
2   limit 1 to english language (2205)
3   limit 2 to meta analysis (14)
4   exp Surgical Procedures, Operative/ (1661433)
5   su.fs. (1152982)

6   exp Postoperative Complications/ (307984)
7   4 or 5 or 6 (2196325)
8   2 not 7 (612)
9   from 8 keep 1-612 (612)

Initial exploratory search strategies for systematic reviews, conducted in January 2007 (postoperative pain was subsequently excluded from the scope):

Acute Pain Management: Postoperative and Inpatient Settings
January 23, 2007

Search strategy 1: PubMed Clinical Queries - Limits; human, English

(pain [mh] AND (drug therapy [sh] OR therapy [sh] OR psychology [sh] OR surgery [sh])) AND systematic[sb]:

((pain,postoperative [mh] OR acute disease [mh]) AND pain measurement [mh]) AND systematic[sb]))

Search strategy 2: PubMed

pain,postoperative [mh] AND evidence-based medicine [mh] AND acute [tw] = 17

Search strategy 3: Cochrane library

Pain management

Pain (and) evidence (and) assessment

Pain in Record Title and management in Record Title and evidence in Record Title in Database of Abstracts of Reviews of Effects

(1-23-07)

 Search strategy 4: PubMed : Acute pain in patients with cognitive impairment or acute psychiatric illness

pain [mh] AND (drug therapy [sh] OR therapy [sh] OR psychology [sh]) AND mental disorders [mh]

Search Strategy 5 - PM Clinical Queries –

pain [mh] AND (drug therapy [sh] OR therapy [sh] OR psychology [sh]) AND mental disorders [mh]

Search strategy 6: PM Clin Quer

(Pain [mh] AND (delirium [tw] OR dementia [tw])) AND systematic[sb]

(1-29-07 – Pubmed)

pain, postoperative [mh] AND (timing [tw] OR assessment [tw]) AND evidence based medicine [mh] = 19

pain measurement [mh] AND evidence based medicine [mh] = 104

March 20, 2007

Ovid search 1

1.pain, postoperative.mp. or Pain, Postoperative/

OR acute disease.mp. or Acute Disease/

AND

patient satisfaction.mp. or Patient Satisfaction/ = 298

Ovid search 2

pain measurement.mp. [mp=title, original title, abstract, name of substance word, subject heading word]

OR

acute disease.mp. [mp=title, original title, abstract, name of substance word, subject heading word]

AND

"Outcome Assessment (Health Care)"/

Ovid search 3 =6

pain, postoperative.mp. or Pain, Postoperative/

AND

patient satisfaction.mp. or Patient Satisfaction/

AND

questionnaires.mp. or Questionnaires/

APPENDIX A, continued. Table of systematic reviews and studies cited, by key question

Title	Conditions	Special populations	KQ1	KQ2	KQ3	KQ4
Acute Pain Management: Scientific Evidence.(1)	Post-operative pain and acute pain in spinal cord injury, burns, cancer, acute zoster, neurological diseases, haematological disorders (e.g. sickle cell disease) HIV/AIDS, renal and biliary colic, musculoskeletal and orofacial pain and headache, phantom limb pain	Elderly, opioid-tolerant patients, patients with obstructive sleep apnea, renal or hepatic impairment or a substance abuse disorder	(2, 3)	(4-18)	(19, 20)	(21-28)
Tools for assessment of pain in nonverbal older adults with dementia: a state-of-the-science review (29)	Types of pain not specified. The assessment scales measured pain by observation of behavioral indicators.	Nonverbal elderly patients with cognitive impairment	--	--	(30-39)	--
Observation scales for pain assessment in older adults with cognitive impairments or communication difficulties (40)	Types of pain not specified. The assessment scales measured pain by observation of behavioral indicators.	Elderly patients with cognitive impairments, communication difficulties, or both.	--	--	(30, 31, 33-35, 37-39, 41-45)	--
Pain in elderly people with severe dementia: a systematic review of behavioural pain assessment tools (46)	Types of pain not specified. The assessment scales measured pain by patient self-report, or behavioral measures.	Elderly patients with cognitive impairment	--	--	(30-33, 37, 38, 47-52)	--
Institutional Approaches to Pain Assessment and Management (2003).(53)	Postoperative pain, non-surgical pain, cancer, HIV disease, sickle cell crisis	--	--	(54-62)	--	--
Do opiates affect the clinical evaluation of patients with acute	Acute abdomen	--	--	(64-72)	--	--

abdominal pain? (63)					
Nonsteroidal anti-inflammatory drugs (NSAIDS) versus opioids for acute renal colic (73)	Acute renal colic pain	--	(74-92)	--	--
Comparing analgesic efficacy of non-steroidal anti-inflammatory drugs given by different routes in acute and chronic pain: a qualitative systematic review (93)	Included 3 trials in renal colic	--	(94-96)	--	--
Hydromorphone for acute and chronic pain (97)	Included one trial in patients with renal colic, and one trial in patients with biliary stone pain.	--	(98, 99)	--	--
Pain management in hospitalized cancer patients: a systematic review (100)	Cancer	--	(101-105)	--	--
Evidence for the optimal management of acute and chronic phantom pain: a systematic review. (5)	Phantom limb pain after amputation	--	(11, 12, 18, 106-114)	--	--

References in Appendix A, Table of Systematic Reviews

1.	Australian and New Zealand College of Anaesthetists and Faculty of Pain Medicine. Acute Pain Management: Scientific Evidence, 2nd edition. Melbourne: Australian and New Zealand College of Anaesthetists. 2005.

2.	Banos JE, Bosch F, Canellas M, Bassols A, Ortega F, Bigorra J. Acceptability of visual analogue scales in the clinical setting: a comparison with verbal rating scales in postoperative pain. Methods & Findings in Experimental & Clinical Pharmacology 1989;11(2):123-7.

3.	Gould TH, Crosby DL, Harmer M, Lloyd SM, Lunn JN, Rees GA, et al. Policy for controlling pain after surgery: effect of sequential changes in management. BMJ 1992;305(6863):1187-93.

4.	Walder B, Schafer M, Henzi I, Tramer MR. Efficacy and safety of patient-controlled opioid analgesia for acute postoperative pain. A quantitative systematic review. Acta Anaesthesiologica Scandinavica 2001;45(7):795-804.

5.	Halbert J, Crotty M. Evidence for the optimal management of acute and chronic phantom pain: a systematic review. Clin J Pain 2002;18(2):84-92.

6.	Bone M, Critchley P, Buggy DJ. Gabapentin in postamputation phantom limb pain: a randomized, double-blind, placebo-controlled, cross-over study. Regional Anesthesia & Pain Medicine 2002;27(5):481-6.

7.	Macintyre PE. Safety and efficacy of patient-controlled analgesia. British Journal of Anaesthesia 2001;87(1):36-46.

8.	Gehling M, Tryba M. [Prophylaxis of phantom pain: is regional analgesia ineffective?]. Schmerz 2003;17(1):11-9.

9.	Dertwinkel R, Henrichs C, Senne I, Tegenthoff M, Weiss T, Malin J, et al. Prevention of severe phantom limb pain by perioperative administration of ketamine - an observational study. Acute Pain 2002;4:9-13.

10.	Hayes C, Armstrong-Brown A, Burstal R. Perioperative intravenous ketamine infusion for the prevention of persistent post-amputation pain: a randomized, controlled trial. Anaesthesia & Intensive Care 2004;32(3):330-8.

11.	Jaeger H, Maier C. Calcitonin in phantom limb pain: a double-blind study. Pain 1992;48(1):21-7.

12.	Nikolajsen L, Hansen CL, Nielsen J, Keller J, Arendt-Nielsen L, Jensen TS. The effect of ketamine on phantom pain: a central neuropathic disorder maintained by peripheral input. Pain 1996;67(1):69-77.

13.	Huse E, Larbig W, Flor H, Birbaumer N. The effect of opioids on phantom limb pain and cortical reorganization. Pain 2001;90(1-2):47-55.

14.	Wu CL, Tella P, Staats PS, Vaslav R, Kazim DA, Wesselmann U, et al. Analgesic effects of intravenous lidocaine and morphine on postamputation pain: a randomized double-blind, active placebo-controlled, crossover trial. Anesthesiology 2002;96(4):841-8.

15.	Flor H, Denke C, Schaefer M, Grusser S. Effect of sensory discrimination training on cortical reorganisation and phantom limb pain. Lancet 2001;357(9270):1763-4.

16.	Sherman RA, Sherman CJ, Gall NG. A survey of current phantom limb pain treatment in the United States. Pain 1980;8:85-99.

17. Lambert A, Dashfield A, Cosgrove C, Wilkins D, Walker A, Ashley S. Randomized prospective study comparing preoperative epidural and intraoperative perineural analgesia for the prevention of postoperative stump and phantom limb pain following major amputation. Regional Anesthesia & Pain Medicine 2001;26(4):316-21.

18. Pinzur MS, Garla PG, Pluth T, Vrbos L. Continuous postoperative infusion of a regional anesthetic after an amputation of the lower extremity. A randomized clinical trial. Journal of Bone & Joint Surgery - American Volume 1996;78(10):1501-5.

19. Chibnall JT, Tait RC. Pain assessment in cognitively impaired and unimpaired older adults: a comparison of four scales. Pain 2001;92(1-2):173-86.

20. Herr KA, Spratt K, Mobily PR, Richardson G. Pain intensity assessment in older adults: use of experimental pain to compare psychometric properties and usability of selected pain scales with younger adults. Clinical Journal of Pain 2004;20(4):207-19.

21. Rapp SE, Ready LB, Nessly ML. Acute pain management in patients with prior opioid consumption: a case-controlled retrospective review. Pain 1995;61(2):195-201.

22. Eilers H, Philip LA, Bickler PE, McKay WR, Schumacher MA. The reversal of fentanyl-induced tolerance by administration of "small-dose" ketamine. Anesthesia & Analgesia 2001;93(1):213-4.

23. Mitra S, Sinatra RS. Perioperative management of acute pain in the opioid-dependent patient. Anesthesiology 2004;101(1):212-27.

24. Wang JK, Nauss LA, Thomas JE. Pain relief by intrathecally applied morphine in man. Anesthesiology 1979;50(2):149-51.

25. de Leon-Casasola OA, Myers DP, Donaparthi S, Bacon DR, Peppriell J, Rempel J, et al. A comparison of postoperative epidural analgesia between patients with chronic cancer taking high doses of oral opioids versus opioid-naive patients. Anesthesia & Analgesia 1993;76(2):302-7.

26. Doverty M, Somogyi AA, White JM, Bochner F, Beare CH, Menelaou A, et al. Methadone maintenance patients are cross-tolerant to the antinociceptive effects of morphine. Pain 2001;93(2):155-63.

27. Bell RF. Low-dose subcutaneous ketamine infusion and morphine tolerance. Pain 1999;83(1):101-3.

28. Sator-Katzenschlager S, Deusch E, Maier P, Spacek A, Kress HG. The long-term antinociceptive effect of intrathecal S(+)-ketamine in a patient with established morphine tolerance. Anesthesia & Analgesia 2001;93(4):1032-4.

29. Herr K, Bjoro K, Decker S. Tools for assessment of pain in nonverbal older adults with dementia: a state-of-the-science review. Journal of Pain & Symptom Management 2006;31(2):170-92.

30. Fuchs-Lacelle S, Hadjistavropoulos T. Development and preliminary validation of the pain assessment checklist for seniors with limited ability to communicate (PACSLAC). Pain Management Nursing 2004;5(1):37-49.

31. Villanueva MR, Smith TL, Erickson JS, Lee AC, Singer CM. Pain Assessment for the Dementing Elderly (PADE): reliability and validity of a new measure. Journal of the American Medical Directors Association 2003;4(1):1-8.

32. Warden V, Hurley AC, Volicer L. Development and psychometric evaluation of the Pain Assessment in Advanced Dementia (PAINAD) scale. Journal of the American Medical Directors Association 2003;4(1):9-15.

33. Abbey J, Piller N, De Bellis A, Esterman A, Parker D, Giles L, et al. The Abbey pain scale: a 1-minute numerical indicator for people with end-stage dementia. International Journal of Palliative Nursing 2004;10(1):6-13.

34. Hurley AC, Volicer BJ, Hanrahan PA, Houde S, Volicer L. Assessment of discomfort in advanced Alzheimer patients. Research in Nursing & Health 1992;15(5):369-77.

35. Lefebvre-Chapiro S, Doloplus Group T. The Doloplus 2 scale - evaluating pain in the elderly. Eur J Palliat Care 2001;8:191-194.

36. Merkel SI, Voepel-Lewis T, Shayevitz JR, Malviya S. The FLACC: a behavioral scale for scoring postoperative pain in young children. Pediatric Nursing 1997;23(3):293-7.

37. Snow AL, Weber JB, O'Malley KJ, Cody M, Beck C, Bruera E, et al. NOPPAIN: a nursing assistant-administered pain assessment instrument for use in dementia. Dementia & Geriatric Cognitive Disorders 2004;17(3):240-6.

38. Feldt KS. The checklist of nonverbal pain indicators (CNPI). Pain Management Nursing 2000;1(1):13-21.

39. Kovach CR, Weissman DE, Griffie J, Matson S, Muchka S. Assessment and treatment of discomfort for people with late-stage dementia. Journal of Pain & Symptom Management 1999;18(6):412-9.

40. van Herk R, van Dijk M, Baar FP, Tibboel D, de Wit R. Observation scales for pain assessment in older adults with cognitive impairments or communication difficulties. Nurs Res 2007;56(1):34-43.

41. Decker SA, Perry AG. The development and testing of the PATCOA to assess pain in confused older adults. Pain Management Nursing 2003;4(2):77-86.

42. Lane P, Kuntupis M, MacDonald S, McCarthy P, Panke JA, Warden V, et al. A pain assessment tool for people with advanced Alzheimer's and other progressive dementias. Home Healthcare Nurse 2003;21(1):32-7.

43. Baker A, Bowring L, Brignell A, Kafford D. Chronic pain management in cognitively impaired patients: a preliminary research project. Perspectives 1996;20(2):4-8.

44. Ekman P, Friesen W. Investigator's guide to the Facial Action Coding System Palo Alto: Consulting Psychologists Press; 1978.

45. Keefe F, Block A. Development of an observation method for assessing pain behavior in chronic low back pain patients. Behavior Therapy 1982;13:363-375.

46. Zwakhalen SMG, Hamers JPH, Abu-Saad HH, Berger MPF. Pain in elderly people with severe dementia: a systematic review of behavioural pain assessment tools. BMC Geriatrics 2006;6:3.

47. Davies E, Male M, Reimer V, Turner M. Pain assessment and cognitive impairment: part 2. Nurs Stand 2004;19(13):33-40.

48. Wary B, Collectief Doloplus. Doloplus-2, une échelle pour évaluer la douleur. Soins Gérontologie 1999;19:25-27.

49. Morello R, Jean A, Alix M. LÉCPA: une échelle comportementale de la douleur pour personnes âgées non communicantes InfoKara 1998;51(3):22-29.

50. Le Quintrec JL, Maga M, Baulon A. L'échelle comportementale simplifiée (E.C.S.). La Revue de Gériatrie 1995;20(6):363-368.

51. Sign B, Orrell M. The development, validity and reliability of a new scale for rating pain in dementia (RaPID). Unpublished manuscript 2003.

52. Simons W, Malabar R. Assessing pain in elderly patients who cannot respond verbally. Journal of Advanced Nursing 1995;22(4):663-9.

53. Merlin T, Hodgkinson B, Macintyre PE, Ludbrook G, Hiller JE. Institutional approaches to pain assessment and management (008PAI). A systematic literature review. Health Technology Assessment Database 2003(1).

54. Miaskowski C, Crews J, Ready LB, Paul SM, Ginsberg B. Anesthesia-based pain services improve the quality of postoperative pain management. Pain 1999;80(1-2):23-9.

55. Benjamin LJ, Swinson GI, Nagel RL. Sickle cell anemia day hospital: an approach for the management of uncomplicated painful crises. Blood 2000;95(4):1130-6.

56. Ahles TA, Seville J, Wasson J, Johnson D, Callahan E, Stukel TA. Panel-based pain management in primary care. a pilot study. Journal of Pain & Symptom Management 2001;22(1):584-90.

57. McQuillar R, Finlay I, Roberts D, Branch C, Forbes K, Spencer MG. The provision of a palliative care service in a teaching hospital and subsequent evaluation of that service. Palliative Medicine 1996;10(3):231-9.

58. Tighe SQ, Bie JA, Nelson RA, Skues MA. The acute pain service: effective or expensive care? Anaesthesia 1998;53(4):397-403.

59. Mackintosh C, Bowles S. Evaluation of a nurse-led acute pain service. Can clinical nurse specialists make a difference? Journal of Advanced Nursing 1997;25(1):30-7.

60. Sartain JB, Barry JJ. The impact of an acute pain service on postoperative pain management. Anaesthesia & Intensive Care 1999;27(4):375-80.

61. Bardiau FM, Braeckman MM, Seidel L, Albert A, Boogaerts JG. Effectiveness of an acute pain service inception in a general hospital. Journal of Clinical Anesthesia 1999;11(7):583-9.

62. Pesut B, Johnson J. Evaluation of an acute pain service. Canadian Journal of Nursing Administration 1997;10(4):86-107.

63. Ranji SR, Goldman LE, Simel DL, Shojania KG. Do opiates affect the clinical evaluation of patients with acute abdominal pain? JAMA 2006;296(14):1764-74.

64. Attard AR, Corlett MJ, Kidner NJ, Leslie AP, Fraser IA. Safety of early pain relief for acute abdominal pain. BMJ 1992;305:554-556.

65. Pace S, Burke T. Intravenous morphine for early pain relief in patients with acute abdominal pain. Academic emergency medicine : official journal of the Society for Academic Emergency Medicine 1996;3(12):1086-92.

66. Mahadevan M, Graff L. Prospective randomized study of analgesic use for ED patients with right lower quadrant abdominal pain. American Journal of Emergency Medicine 2000;18(7):753-6.

67. Attard AR, Corlett MJ, Kidner NJ, Leslie AP, Fraser IA. Safety of early pain relief for acute abdominal pain. BMJ 1992;305(6853):554-6.

68. LoVecchio F, Oster N, Sturmann K, Nelson LS, Flashner S, Finger R. The use of analgesics in patients with acute abdominal pain. Journal of Emergency Medicine 1997;15(6):775-9.

69. Garyfallou GT, Grillo A, O'Connor RE, Fulda GJ, Levine BJ. A controlled trial of fentanyl analgesia in emergency department patients with abdominal pain: can treatment obscure the diagnosis? Acad Emerg Med 1997;4:424.

70. Vermeulen B, Morabia A, Unger PF, Goehring C, Grangier C, Skljarov I, et al. Acute appendicitis: influence of early pain relief on the accuracy of clinical and US findings in the decision to operate--a randomized trial. Radiology 1999;210(3):639-43.

71. Wolfe JM, Smithline HA, Phipen S, Montano G, Garb JL, Fiallo V. Does morphine change the physical examination in patients with acute appendicitis? American Journal of Emergency Medicine 2004;22(4):280-5.

72. Thomas SH, Silen W, Cheema F, Reisner A, Aman S, Goldstein JN, et al. Effects of morphine analgesia on diagnostic accuracy in Emergency Department patients with abdominal pain: a prospective, randomized trial. Journal of the American College of Surgeons 2003;196(1):18-31.

73. Holdgate A, Pollock T. Nonsteroidal anti-inflammatory drugs (NSAIDS) versus opioids for acute renal colic. Cochrane Database of Systematic Reviews 2007(2).

74. Uden P, Rentzhog L, Berger T. A comparative study on the analgesic effects of indomethacin and hydromorphinechloride-atropine in acute, ureteral-stone pain. Acta Chir Scand 1983;149(5):497-9.

75. Quilez C, Perez-Mateo M, Hernandez P, Rubio I. [Usefulness of a non-steroid anti-inflammatory, sodium diclofenac, in the treatment of renal colic. Comparative study with a spasmolytic and an opiate analgesic]. Med Clin (Barc) 1984;82(17):754-5.

76. Lundstam SO, Leissner KH, Wahlander LA, Kral JG. Prostaglandin-synthetase inhibition with diclofenac sodium in treatment of renal colic: comparison with use of a narcotic analgesic. Lancet 1982;1(8281):1096-7.

77. Lehtonen T, Kellokumpu I, Permi J, Sarsila O. Intravenous indomethacin in the treatment of ureteric colic. A clinical multicentre study with pethidine and metamizol as the control preparations. Ann Clin Res 1983;15(5-6):197-9.

78. Persson NH, Bergqvist D, Melander A, Zederfelt B. Comparison of a narcotic (oxicone) and a non-narcotic anti-inflammatory analgesic (indoprofen) in the treatment of renal colic. Acta Chir Scand 1985;151(2):105-8.

79. Hetherington JW, Philp NH. Diclofenac sodium versus pethidine in acute renal colic. Br Med J (Clin Res Ed) 1986;292(6515):237-8.

80. Jonsson PE, Olsson AM, Petersson BA, Johansson K. Intravenous indomethacin and oxycone-papaverine in the treatment of acute renal colic. A double-blind study. Br J Urol 1987;59(5):396-400.

81. Thompson JF, Pike JM, Chumas PD, Rundle JS. Rectal diclofenac compared with pethidine injection in acute renal colic. Bmj 1989;299(6708):1140-1.

82.   Oosterlinck W, Philp NH, Charig C, Gillies G, Hetherington JW, Lloyd J. A double-blind single dose comparison of intramuscular ketorolac tromethamine and pethidine in the treatment of renal colic. J Clin Pharmacol 1990;30(4):336-41.

83.   Arnau JM, Cami J, Garcia-Alonso F, Laporte JR, Palop R. Comparative study of the efficacy of dipyrone, diclofenac sodium and pethidine in acute renal colic. Collaborative Group of the Spanish Society of Clinical Pharmacology. Eur J Clin Pharmacol 1991;40(6):543-6.

84.   Marthak KV, Gokarn AM, Rao AV, Sane SP, Mahanta RK, Sheth RD, et al. A multi-centre comparative study of diclofenac sodium and a dipyrone/spasmolytic combination, and a single-centre comparative study of diclofenac sodium and pethidine in renal colic patients in India. Curr Med Res Opin 1991;12(6):366-73.

85.   Cordell WH, Larson TA, Lingeman JE, Nelson DR, Woods JR, Burns LB, et al. Indomethacin suppositories versus intravenously titrated morphine for the treatment of ureteral colic. Ann Emerg Med 1994;23(2):262-9.

86.   Sandhu DP, Iacovou JW, Fletcher MS, Kaisary AV, Philip NH, Arkell DG. A comparison of intramuscular ketorolac and pethidine in the alleviation of renal colic. Br J Urol 1994;74(6):690-3.

87.   Curry C, Kelly AM. Intravenous tenoxicam for the treatment of renal colic. N Z Med J 1995;108(1001):229-30.

88.   Cordell WH, Wright SW, Wolfson AB, Timerding BL, Maneatis TJ, Lewis RH, et al. Comparison of intravenous ketorolac, meperidine, and both (balanced analgesia) for renal colic. Ann Emerg Med 1996;28(2):151-8.

89.   al-Sahlawi KS, Tawfik OM. Comparative study of the efficacy of lysine acetylsalicylate, indomethacin and pethidine in acute renal colic. Eur J Emerg Med 1996;3(3):183-6.

90.   Larkin GL, Peacock WFt, Pearl SM, Blair GA, D'Amico F. Efficacy of ketorolac tromethamine versus meperidine in the ED treatment of acute renal colic. Am J Emerg Med 1999;17(1):6-10.

91.   Torralba NJA, Montiel RM, Perez BV, Nadal VP, Albacete PM. [Intramuscular ketorolac compared to subcutaneous tramadol in the initial emergency treatment of renal colic]. Arch Esp Urol 1999;52(5):435-7.

92.   Sommer P, Kromann-Andersen B, Lendorf A, Lyngdorf P, Moller P. Analgesic effect and tolerance of Voltaren and Ketogan in acute renal or ureteric colic. Br J Urol 1989;63(1):4-6.

93.   Tramer MR, Williams JE, Carroll D, Wiffen PJ, Moore RA, McQuay HJ. Comparing analgesic efficacy of non-steroidal anti-inflammatory drugs given by different routes in acute and chronic pain: a qualitative systematic review. Acta Anaesthesiologica Scandinavica 1998;42(1):71-9.

94.   Muriel-Villoria C, Zungri-Telo E, Diaz-Curiel M, Fernandez-Guerrero M, Moreno J, Puerta J, et al. Comparison of the onset and duration of the analgesic effect of dipyrone, 1 or 2 g, by the intramuscular or intravenous route, in acute renal colic. European Journal of Clinical Pharmacology 1995;48(2):103-7.

95.   Nelson CE, Nylander C, Olsson AM, Olsson R, Pettersson BA, Wallstrom I. Rectal v. intravenous administration of indomethacin in the treatment of renal colic. Acta Chirurgica Scandinavica 1988;154(4):253-5.

96.   Nissen I, Birke H, Olsen JB, Wurtz E, Lorentzen K, Salomon H, et al. Treatment of ureteric colic. Intravenous versus rectal administration of indomethacin. British Journal of Urology 1990;65(6):576-9.

97.   Quigley C. Hydromorphone for acute and chronic pain. Cochrane Database of Systematic Reviews 2007(2).

98.   Jasani NB, O'Conner RE, Bouzoukis JK. Comparison of hydromorphone and meperidine for ureteral colic. Academic Emergency Medicine 1994;1(6):539-43.

99.   Uden P, Starck CJ, Berger T. Comparison of indomethacin and dihydromorphinone in acute, biliary stone pain. Current Ther Res 1984;36(6):1228-34.

100.   Goldberg GR, Morrison RS. Pain management in hospitalized cancer patients: a systematic review`. J Clin Oncology 2007;25(13):1792-1801.

101.   de Rond ME, de Wit R, van Dam FS, Muller MJ. A Pain Monitoring Program for nurses: effect on the administration of analgesics. Pain 2000;89(1):25-38.

102.   Ward SE, Gordon DB. Patient satisfaction and pain severity as outcomes in pain management: a longitudinal view of one setting's experience. Journal of Pain & Symptom Management 1996;11(4):242-51.

103.   Bookbinder M, Blank AE, Arney E, Wollner D, Lesage P, McHugh M, et al. Improving end-of-life care: development and pilot-test of a clinical pathway. Journal of Pain & Symptom Management 2005;29(6):529-43.

104.   de Rond ME, de Wit R, van Dam FS, Muller MJ. A pain monitoring program for nurses: effects on communication, assessment and documentation of patients' pain. Journal of Pain & Symptom Management 2000;20(6):424-39.

105.   de Rond M, de Wit R, van Dam F. The implementation of a Pain Monitoring Programme for nurses in daily clinical practice: results of a follow-up study in five hospitals. Journal of Advanced Nursing 2001;35(4):590-8.

106.   Bach S, Noreng MF, Tjellden NU. Phantom limb pain in amputees during the first 12 months following limb amputation, after preoperative lumbar epidural blockade. Pain 1988;33(3):297-301.

107.   Lundeberg T. Relief of pain from a phantom limb by peripheral stimulation. Journal of Neurology 1985;232(2):79-82.

108.   Jahangiri M, Jayatunga AP, Bradley JW, Dark CH. Prevention of phantom pain after major lower limb amputation by epidural infusion of diamorphine, clonidine and bupivacaine. Annals of the Royal College of Surgeons of England 1994;76(5):324-6.

109.   Nikolajsen L, Ilkjaer S, Christensen JH, Kroner K, Jensen TS. Randomised trial of epidural bupivacaine and morphine in prevention of stump and phantom pain in lower-limb amputation. Lancet 1997;350(9088):1353-7.

110.   Conine TA, Hershler C, Alexander ST, Crisp R. The efficacy of Farabloc in the treatment of phantom limb pain. Can J Rehabil 1993;6:155-61.

111.   Katz J, Melzack R. Auricular transcutaneous electrical nerve stimulation (TENS) reduces phantom limb pain. Journal of Pain & Symptom Management 1991;6(2):73-83.

112.   Elizaga AM, Smith DG, Sharar SR, Edwards WT, Hansen ST, Jr. Continuous regional analgesia by intraneural block: effect on postoperative opioid

requirements and phantom limb pain following amputation. Journal of Rehabilitation Research & Development 1994;31(3):179-87.

113. Fisher A, Meller Y. Continuous postoperative regional analgesia by nerve sheath block for amputation surgery--a pilot study. Anesthesia & Analgesia 1991;72(3):300-3.

114. Finsen V, Persen L, Lovlien M, Veslegaard EK, Simensen M, Gasvann AK, et al. Transcutaneous electrical nerve stimulation after major amputation. Journal of Bone & Joint Surgery - British Volume 1988;70(1):109-12.

APPENDIX B. Inclusion/exclusion criteria

Code	Include / Exclude	Reason
I1	Include	Published primary research, systematic review, or meta-analysis of studies that a. Were conducted in inpatients with acute pain (including patients with impaired self-report; patients with prexisting opiate therapy; and patients with dependencies on tobacco, alcohol, opioids, or other substances) b. Report data on any of the following i. Association between timing and frequency of pain assessment, severity of pain, and choice of treatment (e.g. regional blocks, medications, or other therapies) ii. Method of pain assessment (e.g. 11-point pain scale, visual analog scale, verbal descriptor scale iii. Timing and route of administration of pain interventions (e.g. oral intermittent pharmacotherapy, intravenous therapy, psychological interventions, positioning, neural blockade, and patient-controlled analgesia); timeliness of enactment of treatment plans, changes in treatment plans iv. Effect of coordination of care with the patient's primary care physician or with a pain consultation service on choice of treatment, clinical outcomes, and safety v. Patient outcomes, including degree of pain relief, pain intensity, emotional well-being, patient satisfaction, physical function, and fitness for rehabilitation of the underlying condition vi. Safety outcomes; severity and frequency of side effects (including somnolence, respiratory depression, confusion, constipation, ileus, vomiting, non-allergic itching, weakness/numbness, and use of naloxone) vii. Length of stay viii. Follow-up of pain
I3	Include	Unpublished research meeting I1 criteria
I4	Include	Non-systematic review or background article meeting I1 criteria
I5	Include	Other (specify)
X1	Exclude	Study outcome does not meet I1 criteria
X2	Exclude	Study population does not meet criteria (e.g. outpatients; inpatients hospitalized 10 days or longer)
X3	Exclude	Type of pain not within scope of review (e.g. post-operative pain, sickle cell disease, cancer pain, chronic pain in patients hospitalized 10 days or longer for whom pain is chronic or refractory)
X4	Exclude	Pain intervention studied is not routinely available in the VA health system
X5	Exclude	Non-English language, no abstract
X6	Exclude	Non-human, animal
X7	Exclude	Other (specify, e.g. off-topic)
X8	Exclude	Wrong study design; no data

APPENDIX C. USPSTF Quality Rating Criteria

Diagnostic Accuracy Studies

Criteria
- Screening test relevant, available for primary care, adequately described
- Study uses a credible reference standard, performed regardless of test results
- Reference standard interpreted independently of screening test
- Handles indeterminate results in a reasonable manner
- Spectrum of patients included in study
- Sample size
- Administration of reliable screening test

Definition of ratings based on above criteria

Good: Evaluates relevant available screening test; uses a credible reference standard; interprets reference standard independently of screening test; reliability of test assessed; has few or handles indeterminate results in a reasonable manner; includes large number (more than 100) broad-spectrum patients with and without disease.

Fair: Evaluates relevant available screening test; uses reasonable although not best standard; interprets reference standard independent of screening test; moderate sample size (50 to 100 subjects) and a "medium" spectrum of patients.

Poor: Has important limitations such as: uses inappropriate reference standard; screening test improperly administered; biased ascertainment of reference standard; very small sample size of very narrow selected spectrum of patients.

Randomized Controlled Trials (RCTs) and Cohort Studies

Criteria
- Initial assembly of comparable groups: RCTs—adequate randomization, including concealment and whether potential confounders were distributed equally among groups; cohort studies—consideration of potential confounders with either restriction or measurement for adjustment in the analysis; consideration of inception cohorts
- Maintenance of comparable groups (includes attrition, cross-overs, adherence, contamination)
- Important differential loss to follow-up or overall high loss to follow-up
- Measurements: equal, reliable, and valid (includes masking of outcome assessment)
- Clear definition of interventions
- Important outcomes considered
- Analysis: adjustment for potential confounders for cohort studies, or intention-to-treat analysis for RCTs (i.e. analysis in which all participants in a trial are analyzed according to the intervention to which they were allocated, regardless of whether or not they completed the intervention)

Definition of ratings based on above criteria

Good: Meets all criteria: Comparable groups are assembled initially and maintained throughout the study (follow-up at least 80 percent); reliable and valid measurement instruments are used and applied equally to the groups; interventions are spelled out clearly; important outcomes are considered; and appropriate attention to confounders in analysis.

Fair: Studies will be graded "fair" if any or all of the following problems occur, without the important limitations noted in the "poor" category below: Generally comparable groups are assembled initially but some question remains whether some (although not major) differences occurred in follow-up; measurement instruments are acceptable (although not the best) and generally applied equally; some but not all important outcomes are considered; and some but not all potential confounders are accounted for.

Poor: Studies will be graded "poor" if any of the following major limitations exists: Groups assembled initially are not close to being comparable or maintained throughout the study; unreliable or invalid measurement instruments are used or not applied at all equally among groups (including not masking outcome assessment); and key confounders are given little or no attention.

Case Control Studies

Criteria
- Accurate ascertainment of cases
- Nonbiased selection of cases/controls with exclusion criteria applied equally to both
- Response rate
- Diagnostic testing procedures applied equally to each group
- Measurement of exposure accurate and applied equally to each group
- Appropriate attention to potential confounding variable

Definition of ratings based on above criteria

Good: Appropriate ascertainment of cases and nonbiased selection of case and control participants; exclusion criteria applied equally to cases and controls; response rate equal to or greater than 80 percent; diagnostic procedures and measurements accurate and applied equally to cases and controls; and appropriate attention to confounding variables.

Fair: Recent, relevant, without major apparent selection or diagnostic work-up bias but with response rate less than 80 percent or attention to some but not all important confounding variables.

Poor: Major selection or diagnostic work-up biases, response rates less than 50 percent, or inattention to confounding variables

Reviewer	Comment	Response	Applies to section of report
Karl Lorenz	Overall, the review provides a helpful summary of clinical questions relevant to expanding pain services, developing standards, and prioritizing a research agenda to improve inpatient pain management in medical settings for veterans. They review found little direct evidence to guide acute pain management in medical inpatients, excluding patients with cancer, those in late life, and the surgical settings.	Noted	General comment
Roger Chou	I think the report does a good job of summarizing the (lack of) evidence for most of the pain management practices in the inpatient setting.	Noted	General comment
Bob Kerns	I am reading with considerable interest this review. One question is puzzling me: I had thought that the review would also include management of pain in surgical settings (note the title of the abstract). Is your intention to provide a separate review with this focus, or did you decide to limit your attention to non surgical, acute medical settings? Or did we simply miscomunicate our intentions?	Regarding the scope, note that before we began the review the ESP committee agreed to a statement that says "Patients with post operative pain, sickle cell disease, and cancer pain, and patients who have been hospitalized 10 days or longer, are excluded."	Scope and key questions
Roger Chou	1) Exclusion of sickle cell patients: I don't remember the justification for excluding sickle cell patients, but it might seem funny to readers/users of the report because sickle cell is probably the population with the most data on pain management in the inpatient setting. I think the reasoning for exclusion should at least be described. Also, it seems a bit inconsistent that evidence on outpatients and cancer pain patients and post op are mentioned in relevant spots but sickle cell evidence is generally not described and is arguably more (or just as) relevant.	See above.	Scope and key questions

APPENDIX D. Reviewer Comments and Responses - VA ESP Acute Pain Management in Inpatients

Reviewer	Comment	Response	Applies to section of report
Karl Lorenz	1. The evidence tables cite about 25 retained studies. 390 studies were reviewed in detail. An accounting of the reasons for exclusion is needed, as well as a summary description of retained studies – overlap and relevance of titles for each question, and a description of the study designs used to answer each question.	This infomation is available upon request.	Results
Karl Lorenz	2. A very brief quantitative summary of the studies included at the beginning of each section would be helpful.	Agree.	Results
Karl Lorenz	3. It is somewhat confusing to have the systematic reviews cited in the text for evidence, but for them to be missing in the tables (which may be used by some readers as the primary source of information). I suggest you include a 'systematic review table' in which you highlight the evidence related to each review (e.g., systematic reviews cited in text for pca as refs 57-66 and so forth) – relevant to each question and note that the current tables are 'other studies' not covered in the reviews (if that's the case).	Agree	Results; evidence tables

Reviewer	Comment	Response	Applies to section of report
Jack Rosenberg	What is obvious is that the search strategy for this may be flawed. Namely, specific disease entities that make up acute non surgical pain were not searched. I also did not see the years of publications that were covered. Much of the literature may be old. Just looking at kidney stone pain for 30 minutes , I pulled these four articles that describe treatment of pain for this entity that are not covered in this review. I did not have the time to go and pull the supporting references. So for a brief synopsis of my opinion, the search for articles should be repeated looking at the questions in reference to particular entities that make up acute pain. for example acute fractures of hip, pelvis, spine)), abdominal, including pancreatic and others. I am also not sure that excluding exacerbations of chronic pain (also called acute on chronic pain) serves us well. There is not much literature on this subject, but these suggestions should help increase the information for analysis.	Our initial searches used broader terms than the specific disease entities; in a supplemental search, using the disease names did not identify additional relevant literature. We alsp conducted a series of supplemental searches relaxing other criteria used in the original searches. These identified 76 potentially relevant abstracts. One of these was a randomized trial of morphine for acute abdominal pain in the emergency room which supported the findings of a systematic review (by Ranji et al) of 12 trials but was too recent to be included in that review. The others concerned clinical settings and conditions that were excluded from our review.	Methods; search strategy
Roger Chou	2) The quality of included studies is summarized in the appendix tables and in the summary table but is not always clear when reading the text. I don't think you need to spend a lot of time describing quality of non RCTS but for RCTS and when describing results of SR's it is probably important to make some mention about quality of the RCTs or studies included in the SR's.	Agree	Results: systematic reviews

APPENDIX D. Reviewer Comments and Responses - VA ESP Acute Pain Management in Inpatients

Reviewer	Comment	Response	Applies to section of report
Roger Chou	3) Regarding KQ #2, some guidelines recommend against use of IM opioid b/c they are equally well absorbed SQ (based on PK data) and this probably should be mentioned at least as background info. Also, there are some old RCTs in cancer pain setttings showing no difference between rectal and oral morphine (Beaver WT 1967 [2 studies]), or IM vs. oral opioids (Babul N 1998 and De Conno F 1995) if you want to describe results from other populations.	This pertains to question 2d. In the section on renal colic we said: "Most evidence about treating renal colic is old and addresses whether to use IM or IV analgesics. The main findings, discussed in more detail below, are (1) NSAIDs provide effective analgesia for acute renal colic, and act more quickly through the IV route than by IM or PR 2) Opioids provide analgesia that is equivalent to NSAIDs but result in a higher incidence of vomiting and other adverse events, particularly pethidine 3) Hydromorphone provided superior pain relief and led to fewer hospital admissions compared with meperidine in one study." We revised this to make the point suggested by the reviewer.	Results: KQ#2
Roger Chou	4) The section on PCA doesn't talk about use of basal infusion + prn versus prn only. My understanding is that some studies suggest that the basal infusion increases opioid use but doesn't improve pain, but I don't have any studies to cite for that. I do think it's a pretty common question on the inpatient setting though, with some people being taught to use basal infusions depending on how much opioid the patient required the previous day etc. Might be worth mentioning as an issue and the evidence (or lack thereof).	This is an important issue clinically, but it is beyond the level of resolution of the literature about nonsurgical pain control. That is, we didn't find any literature about it in the target population.	Results: PCA
Karl Lorenz	Reviewer provided detailed advice for restructuring the future research section (see attached review)	Agree with reorganizing this section using the reviewer's proposed outline.	Future Research Section

Summary Table 1. Studies on methods of pain assessment (KQ1)

Author, Year	Study Design, setting	Sample size	Clinical condition/ baseline pain	Intervention/exposure of interest	Outcomes measured	Results
Carey, 1997[1]	Prospective cohort	267	39.5% acute pain, 40.3% chronic pain. 20.9% reported no pain on admission. Mean for pain intensity ranged from 5.09-5.75.	Patients rated the intensity of pain using each of the 3 scales once over the next 24 hours were also asked which of the scales was easiest to use, whether the scale was helpful or needed further explanation, and employment and education data.	Use of 3 self-rated pain scales; questionnaire also collected demographic information and perceptions about scales.	Patients most frequently selected the VAS faces scale (48.6%), followed by the number scale (35.3%) and line scale (16.1%). None of the demographic variables were associated with preference. Reliability coefficient between scales (Chronbach's alpha) was 0.88. Most (85.8%) patients indicated that a pain rating scale helped them to describe their pain to the nursing staff.
Luger, 2003[2]	Single-site prospective study, convenience sample in Innsbruck, Austria	10 EMS technicians, 10 EMS drivers, 2 ER physicians; 15 trauma patients and 36 nontrauma patients (mostly cardiovascular disease).	15 trauma patients: 7 fractures or lacerations, 5 blunt injuries, 3 penetrating wounds.	Pain assessment was performed at the beginning of emergency care before analgesics, during transport, and upon arrival at the hospital immediately prior to hospitalization.	Severity of pain assessed by patient; EMS physician; EMS technician; EMS driver; at 3 time points (on the scene, during transport, and on arrival at hospital)	The EMS physician underestimate pain 47% of the time; the EMS technician underestimated pain 53% of the time; the EMS driver underestimated pain 57% of the time. The disparity was greatest (60-68%) among patients with severe pain, and lowest (28-36%) among patients with mild pain. The pain intensities on the VAS and VPS were highly correlated (r2=0.86, p=0.0001).
Nelson, 2004[3]	Retrospective cohort study at a suburban university-based ED	521 before the mandatory pain scale; 479 after introducing the pain scale to the ED,	Renal colic, extremity trauma, headache, opthalmologic trauma, or soft tissue injury. Pain varied from 0-10. 8% of patients who reported 0 received analgesia, compared with 74% who reported 9, and 69% who reported 10 as baseline pain.	The standard triage form was revised to include a pain scale in the vital signs section, and the pain assessment was made at triage at the same time as presentation vital signs were assessed. ED staff and patients were not made aware of the study or alerted to the intervention.	1) The proportion of patients who received oral or parenteral analgesia for their pain while in the ED; 2) the time to analgesia administration	The proportion of patients who received analgesia after introduction of the pain scale increased from 25% to 35% (p<0.001). The mean time from triage to analgesia administration was 152 minutes before the intervention, and 113 minutes after (mean difference 39 minutes, 95%CI -7 to 84) but the difference was not statistically significant. Patients with diagnostic uncertainty who received further evaluation were less likely to receive analgesia. 34% who received no workup received analgesia, while only 27% did who underwent a workup (p=0.022). In patients with headache, 23% who underwent CT were treated for pain, whereas 62% of those who did not undergo CT were treated (p<0.001)

APPENDIX E. Evidence Summary Tables

Summary Table 1. Studies on methods of pain assessment (KQ1), continued

Author, Year	Study Design, setting	Sample size	Clinical condition/ baseline pain	Intervention/exposure of interest	Outcomes measured	Results
Morrison, 2006[4]	Controlled clinical trial in an 1171-bed hospital in Mt. Sinai Hospital, New York.	3964 adults	9 medical/surgical units were selected for inclusion based on similar baseline patient demographics and pain scores (3 general medicine, 2 general surgery, 2 specialty surgery, 1 oncology, and 1 mixed oncology/general medicine). 32-38% surgical pts10-16% cancer pts1.5 - 4.8% AIDS pts56% had moderate to complete relief from pain medication29-32% had moderate to severe pain at study enrollment	Education in pain management (months 0-4) was followed by a series of additive 6 to 7-month intervention periods: 1) patient education and nursing pain assessment of current and worst pain, pain relief, and pain acceptability; 2) audit and feedback to nursing staff of patients' pain intensity and staff compliance; and 3) a computerized clinical decision support system (CDSS) to guide analgesic prescribing.	Patients were interviewed within 48 hrs of admission and then once daily. Patients were asked to rate current pain, worst pain over 24 hrs, their pain relief with analgesics, and whether their pain was acceptable to them. Pain and pain relief were rated on 4-pt scales. Outcomes included measures of pain assessment, pain severity, and analgesic prescribing. % of patients who had a daily pain assessment for each shift; % of pts wioth moderate to severe pain 72-96 hrs later, mean pain scores for the first 72 hrs or on postop days 1-3	Pain documentation was improved by >80% using an enhanced pain assessment instrument combined with either audit and feedback or a computerized decision support system. The enhanced pain scale was associated with increased analgesic prescribing.Patients on units using the enhanced pain scale were significantly more likely to have their pain assessed than those on units in which the 1-item pain scale was used (p<0.001). Audit and feedback of pain results was associated with significant increases in pain assessment rates compared with units without audit and feedback (p<0.001). Adding the CSS was associated with significant increases in pain assessment only when compared with units that lacked audit and feedback (p<0.001).Overall the % of pts who received at least 1 pain assessment per day increased from 32.1% with the standard pain assessment to 79.3% when the enhanced pain scale was combined with the CSS, and to more than 80% for interventions using audit and feedback.

Summary Table 2. Studies on the timing and frequency of pain assessment, and timing of treatment (KQ1)

Author, Year	Study Design, setting	Sample size	Clinical condition/ baseline pain	Intervention/ exposure of interest	Outcomes measured	Results
Arendts, 2006 [5]	Retrospective cohort study in an Australian ED	857	Thoracic, including cardiac 12.9%, abdominal 30.6%, urological 11.4%, gynecological 4%, trauma 31%, neurological 35%, and misc. 6.6%. 15% were admitted to critical care, 49% admitted to general ward, and 19% admitted to ED observation	Morphine was the drug used in 94% of cases.	Time from arrival to first dose of opiate. Patients were grouped in 2: time <60 minutes, and time >=60 minutes.	Median time to first dose of opiate = 53 min. 73.5% received no alternative analgesia prior to opiate. Patients with 60+ minute delay were more likely to be female, older, of lower triage acuity, seen by junior medical staff, suffering from nontrauma-related illness, and admitted to hospital rather than discharged. These predictors were significant in multivariate analysis.
Grant, 2006 [6]	Retrospective review of patient records	473	0r 473 pain patients, 213 (45%) had severe pain and 105 (22%) had moderate pain. By type of pain:Chest pain: 14-17%Abdominal pain: 19-21%Headache/neuropathic: 8-11%Muscular: 29-32%Skeletal: 11-15%Ears, nose throat: 2-3%NOS 6-12%	Any form of analgesia	Time intervals between patient arrival, assessment, and delivery of analgesia.	For patients with moderate pain v. severe pain, mean time interval (min):Arrival to doctor assessment: 142 v 42Arrival to prescription of analg: 168 v 58Arrival and receipt of analg: 236 v 72Delay btw prescription and administration of analgesia: 68 v 14.% of patients who received analgesia within time frame meeting BAEM guidelines: 24% in severe pain, 18% in moderate pain. 32% of patients were re-evaluated in terms of analgesia requirements.
Hwang, 2006 [7]	Retrospective review of medical records from a prospective cohort study	158	Patients reporting complaint of pain: 81%	Transfer administrative data (ADT) on time of registration and discharge was used to determine ED crowding risk factors: ED census and mean ED length of stay (LOS) during the hour the index hip fracture patient arrived.	4 quality measures:1) time to pain assessment by a physician;2) documentation of administration of pain medication3) type of analgesic (opioid v nonopioid (NSAID, acetaminophen) if given;4) time to pain treatment	Minutes to first documented pain assessment, mean (range): 40 (0-600)Minutes to first documented pain treatment: 141 (10-525)Delay in treatment, minutes: 122 (0-526)64.1% received analgesia for pain (57% opioids, 7% nonopioids),32.8% of patients for whom opioid was prescribed received meperidine.ED crowding at census levels greater than 120% bed capacity was significantly associated with a lower likelihood of documentation of pain assessment and longer times to pain assessment, in a multivariate analysis that adjusted for age, gender, RAND score, dementia, and mean ED LOS >100% annual.

APPENDIX E. Evidence Summary Tables

Summary Table 2. Studies on the timing and frequency of pain assessment, and timing of treatment (KQ1), continued

Author, Year	Study Design, setting	Sample size	Clinical condition/ baseline pain	Intervention/ exposure of interest	Outcomes measured	Results
Ranji, 2006 [8]	Systematic Review of RCTs of opiate analgesia v placebo in acute abdomen	9 studies in 1062 adults, and 3 studies in 291 children.	3 studies enrolled only patients with right lower quadrant pain; all others enrolled patients with undifferentiated acute abdominal pain.	use of opiate analgesia in acute abdomen	Effect of opiates on patient history (potential to minimize previously concerning symptoms v. increasing its accuracy by calming the patient); on the physical examination; and on potential management errors	11 comparisons from 9 studies in adults showed a trend toward changes in the physical examination with opiate administration, with a summary RR of 1.51 (95%CI 0.85 - 2.69). There was significant heterogeneity among the studies; in 3 comparisons, pain relief reported by the opiate group did not significantly differ from placebo. Studies did not generally distinguish between potentially beneficial changes such as improved localization of tenderness and potentially harmful changes such as changes in peritoneal signs. In 2 studies, loss of periotneal signs after analgesia occurred in 5.6% to 18.7% of patients with opiates, compared with 2.6% to 7.7% of those in the control group. Diagnostic accuracy: a meta-analysis of 4 adult studies indicated no significant change in the rate of incorrect management decisions with opiates vs. placebo. Analgesia was adequate in all these studies, and no significant heterogeneity was found. The frequency of possible unnecessary surgeries was similar between opiate and control groups (7.6% v 7.9%). Meta-analysis showed a non-significant trend toward fewer unnecessary surgeries among patients with opiates.
Shabbir, 2004 [9]	Prospective study in a direct access A&E department where patients were immediately assessed by the surgical on-call service.	100	Acute abdominal pain. Clinical diagnoses included non-specific abdominal pain, PID, peptic ulcer disease, pancreatitis, appendicitis, renal, cholecystitis.	Most common drugs used:diclofenac 37%pethidine 26%Most common routes used:80% intramuscular route0% received intravenous analgesia.	Waiting time for analgesia and its relationship to subjective visual analogue pain scores and clinical diagnoses	Mean waiting time for analgesia was 1.4 hours (range 2 min to 14 hr).Female patients had a longer mean wait time than males (129 min v. 69 min, p=0.09). Patients admitted at nighttime received analgesia quicker (mean 76 min) than during the day time (mean 114 min). 77% were satisfied with the adequacy of analgesia once given; 23% thought the pain relief was not sufficient.Neither clinical diagnosis nor age influenced the timing of analgesia.

Summary Table 2. Studies on the timing and frequency of pain assessment, and timing of treatment (KQ1), continued

Author, Year	Study Design, setting	Sample size	Clinical condition/ baseline pain	Intervention/ exposure of interest	Outcomes measured	Results
Vila, 2005 [10]	Retrospective chart review, single hospital: H.Lee Moffitt Cancer Center and Research Institute	Pre-intervention: 79 opioid ADRs for 117,672 inpatient hospital days, Post-intervention: 67 opioid ADRs for 65,388 inpatient hospital days	Cancer patients	All nursing staff and support personnel were required beginning January 2001 to document each patient's rating of their pain intensity using a numerical scale, along with other vital signs with every routine patient assessment.	Change in patient satisfaction and opioid-related ADRs, including oversedation or respiratory depression requiring discontinuation of th eopioid or reversal with naloxone, in the 4 years before and 2 years after implementation of new pain management standards.	Pre-intervention: 79 opioid ADRs for 117,672 inpatient hospital days, of these 13 involved oversedation. Post-intervention: 67 opioid ADRs for 65,388 inpatient hospital days; of these there were 16 oversedation events.There was a significant increase in the incidence of both events (opioid ADRs and cases of oversedation) post-NPTA ($p=0.01$ and $p=0.03$ respectively). The overall rate of ADRs increased by 49%, with a rate ratio of 1.49 (95%CI 1.08-2.07)67% of patients received analgesia within 1 hour after presentation; approximately 25% waited over 2 hrs.Patient satisfaction ratings increased significantly before and after the NPTA period. ($p<0.00001$)

APPENDIX E. Evidence Summary Tables

Summary Table 3. Studies on the effectiveness and safety of patient-controlled analgesia for acute pain (KQ2)

Author, Year	Study Design, setting	Sample size	Clinical condition/ baseline pain	Intervention/exposure of interest	Results
Evans, 2005[11]	RCT, not placebo-controlled, in an ED	86; 43 in each group	Trauma patients, mostly fracture: 53.4% control, 74% PCA	After baseline measures of VAS, BP, pulse, GCS, SaO2, respiratory rate, an IV cannula was inserted. Controls were given 0-10 mg morphine by IV, titrated by a nurse. Morphine was given at a rate of 1-2 mg/min until by patient's responses pt was comfortable. Pts were then asked to call for further analgesia if needed, and nurse was expected to check pt periodically per ED guidelines. PCA group pts were instructed in the use of the PCA, which administered a 5 mg loading dose with a subsequent bolus dose of 1mg and a lockout interval of 5 minutes. Pain scores and physiological measurements were made at 0, 5, 15, 30, 45, 60, 90, and 120 minutes. Patients were also given 50 mg of cyclizine to minimize nausea and vomiting. Recording of AEs were made by observation. At least 12 hrs after admission to a ward or discharge, patients were contacted by the researcher to complete a satisfaction questionnaire.	The mean pain scores for PCA and controls were similar (4.8 and 4.8, p=0.578). Area under the curve analysis of VAS pain scores confirmed that there was no significant difference between the 2 groups (p=0.784) Twice as much morphine was given to the PCA group, despite the similarity in VAS scores: mean mg PCA v. control: 18.83 v. 7.65. Mean morphine amt delivered over mean time: 7.26 mg/h PCA, 4.03 mg/h control. AEs: PCA patients experienced more events (p ns), most commonly mild sedation. There were no significant differences in the satisfaction questionnaires between the 2 groups.
Fulda, 2005[12]	DB RCT, placebo-controlled	44; 22 in each group	All had thoracic fractures: Unilateral rib fractures = 59% Bilateral rib fractures: 27% The mean injury severity score was 10.5 in the NMS group, 9.8 in the PCA group.	Randomized to 2 groups: nebulized morphine (NMS) or control group (PCA morphine). The PCA group received nebulized saline every 4 hrs with PCA morphine; the NMS group received nebulized morphine every 4 hrs with PCA saline. Pain was considered controlled if VAS <=4 and patient stated pain was well controlled. Patients with uncontrolled pain after 30 minutes Patients in NMS group received additional PRN doses of nebulized morphine every 30 minutes up to 2 treatments, and had the PCA pump adjusted to provide PCA doses of saline every 15 min. Patients in PCA group had PCA delivery adjusted to include addition of 1 mg of morphine every 15 minutes on demand, and received 2 additional PRN nebulized saline treatments every 30 minutes up to 2 treatments	The NMS group required more morphine than the PCA group: the average 4-hr morphine dose was 11.96 for the NMS group, and 6.22 for the PCA group (p<0.001). Although most (74.3%) of observations, patients were alert without evidence of increased sedation, those in the NMS group had lower sedation scores than the PCA group (0.33 v. 0.56, p=0.03). Only 1 patient in the NMS group exceeded sedation level of 1, whereas 5 in the PCA group exceeded this level. However, these 6 patients had less morphine on average than the group as a whole, so there was no correlation. Patients with NMS had a significantly lower mean heart rate, and a non-significantly higher respiratory rate compared with the PCA group. Effect on pain level was similar between NMS and PCA morphine Mean pain score for each group, baseline v. pretreatment v. posttreatment: NMS: 5.38 v. 3.52 v. 2.59, mean overall = 3.38 PCA: 5.73 v. 3.89 v. 2.64, mean overall = 3.84

3/2008

Summary Table 3. Studies on the effectiveness and safety of patient-controlled analgesia for acute pain (KQ2), continued

Author, Year	Study Design, setting	Sample size	Clinical condition/ baseline pain	Intervention/exposure of interest	Results
Moon, 1999[13]	Controlled CT at Univ Cincinnati	34 enrolled; 10 excluded from analysis	Significant thoracic traumatic injury	Epidural analgesia vs. PCA Patients randomized to PCA received a loading dose of IV morphine 0.1 mg/kg before establishment of PCA. The infusion was titrated by a member of the acute pain service to maximize pain relief before handing over the control of the system to the patient. The PCA regimen used morphine 1 mg/ml in bolus doses of 2 mg with a lockout duration of 10 minutes. There was no background infusion. Thoracic epidural catheters were placed by an anesthesiologist in the epidural space between T5 and T7. A 3-ml test dose of lidocaine 1.5% with epinephrine 1:200,000 was then administered through the epidural catheter to exclude subarachnoid or intravascular location of the catheter. Sensory testing of appropriate thoracic dermatomes was performed 10 minutes after to confirm epidural placement of the catheter. The catheter was further dosed with an injection of fentanyl (50 ug) and 3 mg preservative-free morphine. Within 1 hr of placement, a continuous infusion of bupivacaine 0.25% and morphine 0.005% was initiated at a rate of 4-6 ml/hr using an infusion pump. A member of the APS adjusted the infusion rates to optimize pain relief and minimize side effects.	During the first 24 hrs of study, the epidural group had a significant reduction in pain score with coughing, compared with PCA patients. After 48 hrs there was no difference in pain scores btw the 2 routes of opioid administration. On day 3, the epidural group had a 38.7% reduction in pain score compared with the PCA group, whose score was approximately 6.2, the same as for day 2. The epidural group's pain score on day 3 (3.8) was significantly lower than that of the PCA group (p<0.05). PCA patients had a gradual 15% decline in MIF during the study period, whereas the epidural group had a continual increase (23%) By day 3 the epidural group had a significant increase in MIF v. PCA. Tidal volume continually fell for the PCA group (56% on day 3 compared with day 1), but the epidural group had a continual improvement (45% increase from day 1)
Wu, 1999[14]	Retrospective cohort study	64, 32 in each group	Multiple (3+) rib fracture from motor vehicle crash N fractured ribs: 5.6 epidural vs 4.4 PCA (p=0.01) Injury severity score: 21.6 epidural vs 21.9 PCA (p=ns)	Patients who received IV PCA were able to obtain 1 mg of morphine every 6 minutes through the PCA pushbutton. The morphine could be increased by physician order. Epidural catheters were inserted in the thoracic region (T5-T9) with local analgesia (0.125 to 0.25% bupivacaine) and fentanyl (2.5 ug/mL), and the initial infusion rate was 5 to 8ml/h as adjusted by the Acute Pain Service.	There was no difference between PCA and epidural analgesia in duration of analgesia, length of ICU stay, or length of hospital stay. Patients with epidural analgesia had significantly lower pain ratings at all time intervals, with the exception of baseline scores (difference of 0.5 to 1 point higher in the PCA group, p-value ranging from 0.005 to p<0.001 at various time points). There were no differences between the groups with respect to pulmonary, cardiac, or neurologic complications.

APPENDIX E. Evidence Summary Tables

Summary Table 4. Studies on the management of acute pain in renal colic and biliary stone (KQ2)

Author, Year	Study Design, setting	Sample size	Clinical condition/ baseline pain	Intervention/ exposure of interest	Outcomes measured	Results
Holdgate, 2007[15]	Cochrane systematic review, NSAIDs	20 trials with 1613	Most studies included only participants with renal calculi confirmed on subsequent testing, and excluded patients with negative results on followup tests.	Trials compared one of 5 NSAIDS (diclofenac, indomethacin, indoprofen, ketorolac, tenoxicam), to 1 of 7 opioids (pethidine was used in 10 of the 20 trials). The intramuscular route was most commonly used for each drug type (10 trials), followed by the intravenous route (7 trials).	Patient-rated pain and/or time, time to pain relief, need for rescue medication, rate of pain recurrence, adverse events. Major events were defined as GI hemorrhage, renal failure, hypotension, and respiratory depression. Minor adverse events were defined as GI disturbance without bleeding, dizziness, sleepiness.	Patients receiving NSAIDs reported lower pain scores than patients receiving opioids in 10 of 13 studies, though the differences were small. No pooled results on efficacy due to heterogeneity. Use of rescue analgesia was significantly less likely with NSAIDs (RR 0.75, 95%CI 0.61-0.93). More AEs with NSAIDs in the majority of trials, especially vomiting with pethidine. The reviewers concluded that both NSAIDs and opioids provide effective analgesia in acute renal colic, but opioids, particularly pethidine, result in a higher incidence of vomiting and other adverse events.
Jasani, 1994[16]	Prospective DB RCT comparing hydromorphone v. meperidine in a tertiary care center with 93,000 annual ED visits.	36 hydromorphone, 37 meperidine.	Presumed ureteral colic	Comparable doses of the 2 medications were administered at t=0. The patients were randomized to receive either 50 mg meperidine (M) or 1 mg hydromorphone (H) IV in a double-blind manner.	Remedication interval for patients requiring additional analgesia; proportions of men and nonresponders	Baseline VAS pain scores were similar between treatment groups at t=0. The H group had significantly lower pain intensity levels at each timepoint. The M group had significantly more nonresponders than the H group. Significantly fewer patients required IV pyelograms in the H group (28% v 54%, p=0.05) and there were fewer admissions in the H group than the M group (25% v 49%, p=0.08). AEs: there were more patients with nausea and vomiting in the M group compared with H: 40% v 28%, p=0.31. More patients on H had dizziness than did M (22% v 11%, p=0.25. The two groups experienced similar rates of drowsiness (41% H v 46% M).

APPENDIX E. Evidence Summary Tables

Summary Table 4. Studies on the management of acute pain in renal colic and biliary stone (KQ2), continued

Author, Year	Study Design, setting	Sample size	Clinical condition/ baseline pain	Intervention/ exposure of interest	Outcomes measured	Results
Muriel-Villoria, 1995[17]	IM v. IV dipyrone	Varied by intervention, 22-70	Renal colic	dipyrone 1g IM + placebo IV dipyrone 1g IV + placebo IM dipyrone 2g + placebo IM dipyrone 2g + placebo IV diclofenac 75mg IV + placebo IM	Proportion of patients with >50% improvement	Significant differences: dipyrone 2g IV > 1g IV at 10' dicloefenac 75 mg IV > IM at 20' dipyrone 1g IV > 1g IM at 20'
Nelson, 1988[18]	Rectal v. IV indomethacin	Varied by intervention, 53-63	Renal colic	indomethacin 100mg PR indomethacin 50mg IV	VASPI at 10'	IV significantly lower than PR; at 30' no difference. Supplementary analgesics: pr 16/47; IV 8/37
Nissen, 1990[19]	Rectal v. IV indomethacin	Varied by intervention, 44-54	Renal colic	indomethacin 100mg PR indomethacin 50mg IV	VASPI at 10' and 20':	VASPI: IV significantly lower than PR; at 30' no difference. Use of supplementary analgesics: PR 17/63 v. IV 5/53 (p=0.03).
Uden, 1984[20]	Single-blind, randomized trial Biliary stone: subcutaneous injection of dihydromorphinone v. IV indomethacin	42	Acute attacks of biliary stone pain	Group D received 1 mL of dihydromorphinone and patients in Group I received 50 mg of indomethacin intravenously. The surgeon on duty conducted patient exam and provided information about the ongoing study. (Subsequently?) the attendant nurse provided the drug injection, but the examiner was blinded to the treatment. Pain was evaluated at baseline and at 10 and 30 minutes after drug injection. In cases of insufficient pain relief, a second injection was given.	Pain (VAS) at 10 and 30 minutes after administering treatment	N/total free of pain at 10 minutes and 30 minutes: Group D: 2/21 at 10 min, 11/21 at 30 min Group I: 2/21 at 10 min, 10/21 at 30 min Mean scores at baseline, 10 minutes, and 30 minutes: Group D: 71.8, 44.1, 14.2 Group I: 68.5, 32.4, 15.8 Pain reduction within each group was statistically significant (p<0.01) whereas the difference between the two groups was not. AEs: 2 pts in each group felt nausea and vertigo. 1 in D developed a red, itching subcutaneous infiltration at injection site. 1 in Group I vomited during injection, another in Group I experienced nasal congestion.

APPENDIX E. Evidence Summary Tables

Summary Table 5. Studies on the effectiveness and safety of neural blockade for acute pain (KQ2)

Author, Year	Study Design, setting	Sample size	Clinical category; baseline pain	Intervention/exposure of interest	Outcomes measured	Results
Chudinov, 1999[21]	Randomized trial in orthopedic hospital, Israel	40	Hip fracture, undergoing surgery	Psoas compartment block using 2mg/kg/body weight of 0.25% bupivacaine with adrenaline (0.8 ml/kg) and supplementary doses as required via catheter vs. no block	Length of follow-up: perioperative period only (72 hours). Pain relief assessed by VAS. Adverse effects of the block	The psoas compartment block resulted in significantly less pain at 8 and 16 hours pre-operatively, and also at 16, 24, and 32 hours post-operatively. Proportionally more patients who received the psoas block were satisfied with pain control compared with controls.
Haddad, 1995[22]	Randomised trial	50	Extracap-sular hip fracture	Femoral nerve block inserted at time of admission using 0.3ml/kg of 0.25% buipivacaine vs. control group (no injection	Mean pain score using VAS: pre-block and at 15 mins, 2 hrs and 8 hrs. Amount of analgesic administration within first 24 hrs of co-codramol, voltarol, pethidine. Incidence of respiratory infections, CVA, pulmonary embolism, deep vein thrombosis, urinary tract infection, skin breakdown, mortality, failed nerve block.	Femoral nerve block provided a greater reduction in the mean pain scores that was statistically significant at 15 minutes (mean change -2.6 v. -0.7) and at 2 hours (mean reduction -3.0 v. -1.2). The number of parenteral analgesic drugs administered in the 24 hrs from admission was reduced for the nerve block group. Local or systemic complications did not occur with the use of femoral nerve blocks.
Scheinin, 2000[23]	Randomized trial, orthopedic hospital in Finland	59	Hip fracture, undergoing surgery	Lumbar epidural using bupivacaine and fentanyl inserted within 6 hrs of admission. Infusion rate adjusted according to patients requirements vs intramuscular opiate (oxycodone 0.1-0.15mg/kg) at 6 hourly intervals as necessary. All patients operated on using spinal anesthesia	Length of follow-up for clinical outcomes was 3 days. Mortality for 3 years was determined using central statistic register. Pain relief as assessed by VAS (scale 0-100). Ischemic episodes as determined by continuous electrocardiogram recording; nocturnal oxygen saturation; itching; nausea; quality of sleep; mortality.	Pre-operative pain scores did not significantly differ (p=0.42) continuous epidural infusion of bupivacaine plus fentanyl (mean value 34) vs controls who received parenteral opiates IM (mean 42), although post-operative pain scores were significantly (p=0.006) reduced in the epidural group (mean 22) compared with intramuscular opiates (mean 35). No mention of complications specific to the treatment.

Summary Table 5. Studies on the effectiveness and safety of neural blockade for acute pain (KQ2), continued

Author, Year	Study Design, setting	Sample size	Clinical condition/ baseline pain	Intervention/exposure of interest	Outcomes measured	Results
Halbert, 2002 #1428[24]	SR of 12 controlled trials that reported phantom pain as an outcome	Included 12 trials, total 375 patients (both men and women), ages 47-75.	8 trials of treatment of acute phantom pain with preoperative, intra-operative, and early (<2 weeks) postoperative interventions	8 trials on phantom limb pain studied epidural treatments (3 trials); regional nerve blocks (3); calcitonin (1); and transcutaenous electrical nerve stimulation (1). 4 trials on late postoperative pain studied transcutaneous electrical nerve stimulation (2) and Farablock (a metal threaded sock) and ketamine (1 trial each). In 8 preop/intraop/early post-op trials, the interventions included epidural anesthesia (3 trials), regional nerve blocks (3), intravenous calcitonin (1) and TENS. Controls received a placebo consisting of a saline infusion or epidural anesthesia consisting of on-demand opioid analgesia. 5 trials used opioid analgesia, and 1 trial used sham TENS with and without chlorpromazine. Trials that used epidural anesthesia commenced 18-72 hours before surgery. Blockade anesthesia commenced during the operation or postoperatively. 4 trials of late postop interventions included TENS, Farabloc, vibratory stimulation, and infused ketamine.	Effect on phantom limb pain at various time points up to 12 months post-amputation	Up to 70% of patients have phantom limb pain after amputation. There is little evidence from randomized trials to guide clinicans with treatment. Evidence on preemptive epidurals, early regional nerve blocks, and mechanical vibratory stimulation provides inconsistent support for these treatments.

APPENDIX E. Evidence Summary Tables

Summary Table 5. Studies on the effectiveness and safety of neural blockade for acute pain (KQ2), continued

Author, Year	Study Design, setting	Sample size	Clinical condition/ baseline pain	Intervention/exposure of interest	Outcomes measured	Results
Knoop, 1994[25]	Randomized prospective, nonblinded clinical study, convenience sample; inner-city and community hospital ER	30	Patients had 3rd or 4th finger injuries including and distal to the proximalinterp halangeal joint that required digital anesthesia. Injuries included lacerations (67%) and infections (27%).	Digital blocks and a metacarpal block were performed on each patient, in randomized order. Additional anesthesia was given and noted when required for all patients. After a period of no less than 10 minutes, the patient was treated in a mannger consistent with the injury (ie, sutures, incision, and drainage).	Patients immediately rated pain associated with each technique on a nonsegmented VAS. Efficacy was assessed by requirement for additional anesthesia and anesthesia to pinprick. Time to anesthesia was assessed after each block in 23 patients. Patients were asked which technique they thought was more painful or if there was no difference between the 2 techniques. Responses were recorded for 10 minutes.	Digital block was less painful than metacarpal block by both VAS and by verbal comparison, but the differences did not reach statistical significance. There were no sig. Diffs in the VAS scores of the first block compared with the second block. Mean VAS scores were 2.53 cm for digital block, and 3.35 cm for metacarpal block (p=ns). 40% of patients rated the digital block as more painful, and 7% noted no difference in pain between the blocks (p=ns). Digital block was found to be more efficacious as metacarpal block failed anesthesia to pinprick in seven of 30 metacarpol blocks (23%) compared with one of 30 (3%) for digital block (p=0.02). When requirement for additional anesthesia was assessed, digital block was adequate 97% of the time (29 of 30 blocks), while metacarpal block was adequate 87% of the time (26 of 30 blocks, p=ns). Time to anesthesia available in 23 patients was found to be significantly shorter for digital block compared with metacarpal block, with a mean of 2.82 minutes vs. 6.35 minutes (p<0.0001).

APPENDIX E. Evidence Summary Tables

References in Appendix E, Evidence Summary Tables

1. Carey SJ, Turpin C, Smith J, Whatley J, Haddox D. Improving pain management in an acute care setting. The Crawford Long Hospital of Emory University experience. *Orthopaedic Nursing.* Jul-Aug 1997;16(4):29-36.

2. Luger TJ, Lederer W, Gassner M, Lockinger A, Ulmer H, Lorenz IH. Acute pain is underassessed in out-of-hospital emergencies. *Academic Emergency Medicine.* Jun 2003;10(6):627-632.

3. Nelson BP, Cohen D, Lander O, Crawford N, Viccellio AW, Singer AJ. Mandated pain scales improve frequency of ED analgesic administration. *American Journal of Emergency Medicine.* Nov 2004;22(7):582-585.

4. Morrison RS, Meier DE, Fischberg D, et al. Improving the management of pain in hospitalized adults. *Archives of Internal Medicine.* May 8 2006;166(9):1033-1039.

5. Arendts G, Fry M. Factors associated with delay to opiate analgesia in emergency departments. *Journal of Pain.* Sep 2006;7(9):682-686.

6. Grant PS. Analgesia delivery in the ED. *American Journal of Emergency Medicine.* Nov 2006;24(7):806-809.

7. Hwang U, Richardson LD, Sonuyi TO, Morrison RS. The effect of emergency department crowding on the management of pain in older adults with hip fracture. *Journal of the American Geriatrics Society.* Feb 2006;54(2):270-275.

8. Ranji SR, Goldman LE, Simel DL, Shojania KG. Do opiates affect the clinical evaluation of patients with acute abdominal pain? *JAMA.* Oct 11 2006;296(14):1764-1774.

9. Shabbir J, Ridgway PF, Lynch K, et al. Administration of analgesia for acute abdominal pain sufferers in the accident and emergency setting. *European Journal of Emergency Medicine.* Dec 2004;11(6):309-312.

10. Vila H, Jr., Smith RA, Augustyniak MJ, et al. The Efficacy and Safety of Pain Management Before and After Implementation of Hospital-Wide Pain Management Standards: Is Patient Safety Compromised by Treatment Based Solely on Numerical Pain Ratings? *Anesth. Analg.* August 1, 2005 2005;101(2):474-480.

11. Evans E, Turley N, Robinson N, Clancy M. Randomised controlled trial of patient controlled analgesia compared with nurse delivered analgesia in an emergency department. *Emergency Medicine Journal.* Jan 2005;22(1):25-29.

12. Fulda GJ, Giberson F, Fagraeus L. A prospective randomized trial of nebulized morphine compared with patient-controlled analgesia morphine in the management of acute thoracic pain. *Journal of Trauma-Injury Infection & Critical Care.* Aug 2005;59(2):383-388; discussion 389-390.

13. Moon MR, Luchette FA, Gibson SW, et al. Prospective, randomized comparison of epidural versus parenteral opioid analgesia in thoracic trauma. *Annals of Surgery.* May 1999;229(5):684-691; discussion 691-682.

14. Wu CL, Jani ND, Perkins FM, Barquist E. Thoracic epidural analgesia versus intravenous patient-controlled analgesia for the treatment of rib fracture pain after motor vehicle crash. *Journal of Trauma-Injury Infection & Critical Care.* Sep 1999;47(3):564-567.

15. Holdgate A, Pollock T. Nonsteroidal anti-inflammatory drugs (NSAIDS) versus opioids for acute renal colic [Systematic Review]. *Cochrane Database of Systematic Reviews.* 2007(2).

16. Jasani NB, O'Conner RE, Bouzoukis JK. Comparison of hydromorphone and meperidine for ureteral colic. *Academic Emergency Medicine.* Nov-Dec 1994;1(6):539-543.

APPENDIX E. Evidence Summary Tables

17.   Muriel-Villoria C, Zungri-Telo E, Diaz-Curiel M, et al. Comparison of the onset and duration of the analgesic effect of dipyrone, 1 or 2 g, by the intramuscular or intravenous route, in acute renal colic. *European Journal of Clinical Pharmacology.* 1995;48(2):103-107.

18.   Nelson CE, Nylander C, Olsson AM, Olsson R, Pettersson BA, Wallstrom I. Rectal v. intravenous administration of indomethacin in the treatment of renal colic. *Acta Chirurgica Scandinavica.* Apr 1988;154(4):253-255.

19.   Nissen I, Birke H, Olsen JB, et al. Treatment of ureteric colic. Intravenous versus rectal administration of indomethacin. *British Journal of Urology.* Jun 1990;65(6):576-579.

20.   Uden P, Starck CJ, Berger T. Comparison of indomethacin and dihydromorphinone in acute, biliary stone pain. *Current Ther Res.* 1984;36(6):1228-1234.

21.   Chudinov A, Berkenstadt H, Salai M, Cahana A, Perel A. Continuous psoas compartment block for anesthesia and perioperative analgesia in patients with hip fractures. *Regional Anesthesia & Pain Medicine.* Nov-Dec 1999;24(6):563-568.

22.   Haddad FS, Williams RL. Femoral nerve block in extracapsular femoral neck fractures. *Journal of Bone & Joint Surgery - British Volume.* Nov 1995;77(6):922-923.

23.   Scheinin H, Virtanen T, Kentala E, et al. Epidural infusion of bupivacaine and fentanyl reduces perioperative myocardial ischaemia in elderly patients with hip fracture--a randomized controlled trial. *Acta Anaesthesiologica Scandinavica.* Oct 2000;44(9):1061-1070.

24.   Halbert J, Crotty M. Evidence for the optimal management of acute and chronic phantom pain: a systematic review. *Clin J Pain* 2002;18(2):84-92.

25.   Knoop K, Trott A, Syverud S. Comparison of digital versus metacarpal blocks for repair of finger injuries. *Annals of Emergency Medicine.* Jun 1994;23(6):1296-1300.

www.ingramcontent.com/pod-product-compliance
Lightning Source LLC
Chambersburg PA
CBHW081552170526
45166CB00009B/2672